CANCER ETIOLOGY, DIAGNOSIS AND TREATMENTS

COPING WITH CANCER

PAIN CONTROL AND EATING SUGGESTIONS

CANCER ETIOLOGY, DIAGNOSIS AND TREATMENTS

Additional books in this series can be found on Nova's website under the Series tab.

Additional e-books in this series can be found on Nova's website under the e-book tab.

CANCER ETIOLOGY, DIAGNOSIS AND TREATMENTS

COPING WITH CANCER

PAIN CONTROL AND EATING SUGGESTIONS

EDWARD H. GINN
EDITOR

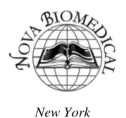

New York

Copyright © 2014 by Nova Science Publishers, Inc.

All rights reserved. No part of this book may be reproduced, stored in a retrieval system or transmitted in any form or by any means: electronic, electrostatic, magnetic, tape, mechanical photocopying, recording or otherwise without the written permission of the Publisher.

For permission to use material from this book please contact us:
Telephone 631-231-7269; Fax 631-231-8175
Web Site: http://www.novapublishers.com

NOTICE TO THE READER

The Publisher has taken reasonable care in the preparation of this book, but makes no expressed or implied warranty of any kind and assumes no responsibility for any errors or omissions. No liability is assumed for incidental or consequential damages in connection with or arising out of information contained in this book. The Publisher shall not be liable for any special, consequential, or exemplary damages resulting, in whole or in part, from the readers' use of, or reliance upon, this material. Any parts of this book based on government reports are so indicated and copyright is claimed for those parts to the extent applicable to compilations of such works.

Independent verification should be sought for any data, advice or recommendations contained in this book. In addition, no responsibility is assumed by the publisher for any injury and/or damage to persons or property arising from any methods, products, instructions, ideas or otherwise contained in this publication.

This publication is designed to provide accurate and authoritative information with regard to the subject matter covered herein. It is sold with the clear understanding that the Publisher is not engaged in rendering legal or any other professional services. If legal or any other expert assistance is required, the services of a competent person should be sought. FROM A DECLARATION OF PARTICIPANTS JOINTLY ADOPTED BY A COMMITTEE OF THE AMERICAN BAR ASSOCIATION AND A COMMITTEE OF PUBLISHERS.

Additional color graphics may be available in the e-book version of this book.

Library of Congress Cataloging-in-Publication Data

ISBN: 978-1-63321-039-4

Published by Nova Science Publishers, Inc. † New York

CONTENTS

Preface vii

Chapter 1 Pain Control: Support for People with Cancer 1
National Cancer Institute

Chapter 2 Eating Hints:
Before, During, and After Cancer Treatment 45
National Cancer Institute

Index 99

PREFACE

People who have cancer don't always have pain. Everyone is different. But if an individual does have cancer pain, it can almost always be relieved. Cancer pain can range from mild to very severe. Some days it can be worse than others. It can be caused by the cancer itself, the treatment, or both. This book discusses pain control medicines and other methods to help manage pain, and addresses the physical and emotional effects of pain. It includes questions to ask health care professionals, a sample pain control record, a list of resources, and a glossary of terms. This book also provides information and recipes to help patients meet their needs for good nutrition during cancer treatment.

Chapter 1 - Having cancer doesn't mean that you'll have pain. But if you do, you can manage most of your pain with medicine and other treatments.

This chapter will show you how to work with your doctors, nurses, and others to find the best way to control your pain. It will discuss causes of pain, medicines, how to talk to your doctor, and other topics that may help you.

Chapter 2 - Eating Hints is written for you—someone who is about to get, or is now getting, cancer treatment. Your family, friends, and others close to you may also want to read this chapter.

You can use this chapter before, during, and after cancer treatment. It has hints about common types of eating problems, along with ways to manage them.

This chapter covers:

- What you should know about cancer treatment, eating well, and eating problems
- How feelings can affect appetite

- Hints to manage eating problems
- How to eat well after cancer treatment ends
- Foods and drinks to help with certain eating problems
- Ways to learn more

Talk with your doctor, nurse, or dietitian about any eating problems that might affect you during cancer treatment. He or she may suggest that you read certain sections or follow some of the tips.

In: Coping With Cancer
Editor: Edward H. Ginn

ISBN: 978-1-63321-039-4
© 2014 Nova Science Publishers, Inc.

Chapter 1

PAIN CONTROL: SUPPORT FOR PEOPLE WITH CANCER[*]

National Cancer Institute

CANCER PAIN CAN BE MANAGED

Having cancer doesn't mean that you'll have pain. But if you do, you can manage most of your pain with medicine and other treatments.

This chapter will show you how to work with your doctors, nurses, and others to find the best way to control your pain. It will discuss causes of pain, medicines, how to talk to your doctor, and other topics that may help you.

YOUR "HEALTH CARE TEAM" CAN HELP YOU MANAGE CANCER PAIN

In this chapter, your "health care team" can mean any of the professionals you see as part of your medical care. These may include your **oncologist**, your family doctor, nurses, physical therapists, pharmacists, oncology social workers, clergy members, and others.

---

[*] This is an edited, reformatted and augmented version of National Institutes of Health Publication No. 12-6287, revised July 2012.

READ WHAT YOU NEED

Use this chapter in the way that works best for you. You may read it from front to back. Or you may want to read different parts as you need them.

There is a list of resources toward the end of the chapter.

Words in bold are explained at the end of the chapter in "Words To Know." They include terms you might hear in doctors' offices or hospitals.

1. WHAT YOU SHOULD KNOW ABOUT TREATING CANCER PAIN

You Don't Have to Accept Pain

People who have cancer don't always have pain. Everyone is different. But if you do have cancer pain, you should know that you don't have to accept it. Cancer pain can almost always be relieved.

The key messages we want you to learn from this chapter are:

- Your pain *can* be managed.
- Controlling pain *is part* of your cancer treatment.
- Talking openly with your doctor and health care team will help them manage your pain.
- The best way to control pain is to stop it from starting or keep it from getting worse.
- There are many different medicines to control pain. Everyone's pain control plan is different.
- Keeping a record of your pain will help create the best pain control plan for you.
- People who take cancer pain medicines as prescribed rarely become addicted to them.
- Your body does *not* become immune to pain medicine. Stronger medicines should not be saved for "later."

Palliative Care and Pain Specialists Can Help

Cancer pain can be reduced so that you can enjoy your normal routines and sleep better. It may help to talk with a palliative care or pain specialist. These may be oncologists, *anesthesiologists*, *neurologists*, surgeons, other doctors, nurses, or pharmacists. If you have a pain control team, it may also include psychologists and social workers.

Pain and *palliative care* specialists are experts in pain control. Palliative care specialists treat the symptoms, *side effects*, and emotional problems of both cancer and its treatment. They will work with you to find the best way to manage your pain. Ask your doctor or nurse to suggest someone. Or contact one of the following for help finding a specialist in your area:

- Cancer center
- Your local hospital or medical center
- Your primary care provider
- People who belong to pain support groups in your area
- The Center to Advance Palliative Care, http://www.getpalliativecare.org (for lists of providers in each state)

When cancer pain *is not treated* properly, you may be:

- Tired
- Depressed
- Angry
- Worried
- Lonely
- Stressed

When cancer pain *is managed* properly, you can:

- Enjoy being active
- Sleep better
- Enjoy family and friends
- Improve your appetite
- Enjoy sexual intimacy
- Prevent depression

2. TYPES AND CAUSES OF CANCER PAIN

Cancer pain can range from mild to very severe. Some days it can be worse than others. It can be caused by the cancer itself, the treatment, or both.

You may also have pain that has nothing to do with your cancer. Some people have other health issues or headaches and muscle strains. But always check with your doctor before taking any over-the-counter medicine to relieve everyday aches and pains. This will help ensure that there will be no interactions with other drugs or safety concerns to know about.

Different Types of Pain

Here are the common terms used to describe different types of pain:

- *Acute pain* ranges from mild to severe. It comes on quickly and lasts a short time.
- *Chronic pain* ranges from mild to severe. It either won't go away or comes back often.
- *Breakthrough pain* is an intense rise in pain that occurs suddenly or is felt for a short time. It can occur by itself or in relation to a certain activity. It may happen several times a day, even when you're taking the right dose of medicine. For example, it may happen as the current dose of your medicine is wearing off.

What Causes Cancer Pain?

Cancer and its treatment cause most cancer pain. Major causes of pain include:

- **Pain from medical tests**: Some methods used to diagnose cancer or see how well treatment is working are painful. Examples may be a biopsy, spinal tap, or bone marrow test. If you are told you need the procedure, don't let concerns about pain stop you from having it done. Talk with your doctor ahead of time about what will be done to lessen any pain you may have.
- **Pain from a tumor**: If the cancer grows bigger or spreads, it can cause pain by pressing on the tissues around it. For example, a tumor

can cause pain if it presses on bones, nerves, the spinal cord, or body organs.
- **Spinal cord compression**: When a tumor spreads to the spine, it can press on the spinal cord and cause spinal cord compression. The first sign of this is often back or neck pain, or both. Coughing, sneezing, or other motions may make it worse.
- **Pain from treatment**: *Chemotherapy, radiation therapy*, surgery, and other treatments may cause pain for some people. Some examples of pain from treatment are:
  - **Neuropathic pain**: This is pain that may occur if treatment damages the nerves. The pain is often burning, sharp, or shooting. The cancer itself can also cause this kind of pain.
  - **Phantom pain**: You may still feel pain or other discomfort coming from a body part that has been removed by surgery. Doctors aren't sure why this happens, but it's real.

How much pain you feel depends on different things. These include where the cancer is in your body, what kind of damage it is causing, and how you experience the pain in your body. Everyone is different.

Call Your Doctors Right Away

Listen to your body. If you notice that everyday actions, such as coughing, sneezing, moving, walking, or standing, suddenly cause new pain or your pain to get worse, tell your doctors right away. Also let them know if you have unusual rashes or bowel or bladder changes.

3. TALKING ABOUT YOUR PAIN

Pain Control Is Part of Treatment. Talking Openly Is Key

> "At first I tried to be brave. Now I realize that the only way to handle my pain is to be open and honest about it with my health care team. It's the only way I can stay on top of it and keep it under control." — Janie

Controlling Pain Is a Key Part of Your Overall Cancer Treatment

The most important member of the team is you. You're the only one who knows what your pain feels like. Talking about pain is important. It gives your health care team the feedback they need to help you feel better.

Some people with cancer don't want to talk about their pain. They think that they'll distract their doctors from working on ways to help treat their cancer. Or they worry that they won't be seen as "good" patients. They also worry that they won't be able to afford pain medicine. As a result, people sometimes get so used to living with their pain that they forget what it's like to live without it.

But your health care team needs to know details about your pain and whether it's getting worse. This helps them understand how the cancer and its treatment are affecting your body. And it helps them figure out how to best control the pain.

Try to talk openly about any other medical problems and fears you have. And if money worries are stopping you, be sure to read the Financial Issues section later in this chapter. There may be ways to help you get the medicine you need.

Tell your health care team if you're:

- Taking any medicine to treat other health problems
- Taking more or less of the pain medicine than prescribed
- Allergic to certain drugs
- Using any over-the-counter medicines, home remedies, or herbal or alternative therapies

This information could affect the pain control plan your doctor suggests for you. If you feel uneasy talking about your pain, bring a family member or friend to speak for you. Or let your loved one take notes and ask questions. Remember, open communication between you, your loved ones, and your health care team will lead to better pain control.

Talking About Your Pain

The first step in getting your pain under control is talking honestly about it. Try to talk with your health care team and your loved ones about what you are feeling. This means telling them:

- Where you have pain
- What it feels like (sharp, dull, throbbing, constant, burning, or shooting)
- How strong your pain is
- How long it lasts
- What lessens your pain or makes it worse
- When it happens (what time of day, what you're doing, and what's going on)
- If it gets in the way of daily activities

Describe and Rate Your Pain

You will be asked to describe and rate your pain. This provides a way to assess your *pain threshold* and measure how well your pain control plan is working.

Your doctor may ask you to describe your pain in a number of ways. A pain scale is the most common way. The scale uses the numbers 0 to 10, where 0 is no pain, and 10 is the worst. You can also use words to describe pain, like pinching, stinging, or aching. Some doctors show their patients a series of faces and ask them to point to the face that best describes how they feel.

No matter how you or your doctor keep track of your pain, make sure that you do it the same way each time. You also need to talk about any new pain you feel.

It may help to keep a record of your pain. Some people use a pain diary or journal. Others create a list or a computer spreadsheet. Choose the way that works best for you.

Your record could list:

- When you take pain medicine
- Name and dose of the medicine you're taking
- Any side effects you have
- How much the medicine lowers the pain level
- How long the pain medicine works
- Other pain relief methods you use to control your pain
- Any activity that is affected by pain, or makes it better or worse
- Things that you can't do at all because of the pain

Share your record with your health care team. It can help them figure out how helpful your pain medicines are, or if they need to change your pain control plan.

Here are some ways your health care team may ask you to describe or rate your pain:

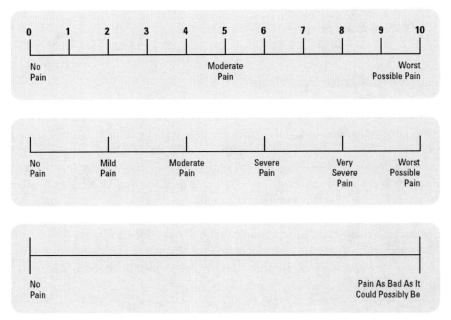

0–10 Numeric Pain Intensity Scale, Simple Descriptive Pain Intensity Scale, and Visual Analog Scale (VAS): Acute Pain Management Guideline Panel. Acute Pain Management in Adults: Operative Procedures. Quick Reference Guide for Clinicians AHCPR Pub. No. 92-0019. Rockville, MD: Agency for Health Care Policy and Research, Public Health Service, U.S. Department of Health and Human Services.

Share Your Beliefs

Some people don't want to take medicine, even when it's prescribed by the doctor. Taking it may be against religious or cultural beliefs. Or there may be other personal reasons why someone won't take medicine. If you feel any of these ways about pain medicine, it's important to share your views with your health care team. If you prefer, ask a friend or family member to share them for you. Talking openly about your beliefs will help your health care team find a plan that works best for you.

"It makes sense. If you don't tell someone about your pain, then no one can help you! And the pain won't go away by itself." — Joe

4. YOUR PAIN CONTROL PLAN

"It took a few visits to my health care team to get my pain under control. But by trying different medicines and doses, I now have a pain plan that works for me." — Michelle

Make Your Pain Control Plan Work for You

Your pain control plan will be designed for you and your body. Everyone has a different pain control plan. Even if you have the same type of cancer as someone else, your plan may be different.

Take your pain medicine dose on schedule to keep the pain from starting or getting worse. This is one of the best ways to stay on top of your pain. Don't skip doses. Once you feel pain, it's harder to control and may take longer to get better.

Here are some other things you can do:

- Bring your list of medicines to each visit.
- If you are seeing more than one doctor, make sure each one sees your list of medicines, especially if he or she is going to change or prescribe medicine.
- Never take someone else's medicine. What helped a friend or relative may not help you. Do not get medicine from other countries or the Internet without telling your doctor.
- Don't wait for the pain to get worse.
- Ask your doctor to change your pain control plan if it isn't working.

The Best Way to Control Pain Is to Stop It before It Starts or Prevent It from Getting Worse

Don't wait until the pain gets bad or unbearable before taking your medicine. Pain is easier to control when it's mild. And you need to take pain medicine often enough to stay ahead of your pain. Follow the dose schedule your doctor gives you. Don't try to "hold off" between doses. If you wait:

- Your pain could get worse.
- It may take longer for the pain to get better or go away.
- You may need larger doses to bring the pain under control.

Keep a List of All Your Medicines

Make a list of all the medicines you are taking. If you need to, ask a member of your family or health care team to help you. *Bring this list of medicines to each visit.* You can take most pain medicines with other *prescription* drugs. But your health care team needs to know what you take and when. Tell them each drug you are taking, no matter how harmless you think it might be. Even over-the-counter medicines, herbs, and *supplements* can interfere with cancer treatment. Or they could cause serious side effects or reactions.

How to Tell When You Need a New Pain Control Plan

Here are a few things to watch out for and tell your health care team about:

- Your pain isn't getting better or going away.
- Your pain medicine doesn't work as long as your doctor said it would.
- You have breakthrough pain.
- You have side effects that don't go away.
- Pain interferes with things like eating, sleeping, or working.
- The schedule or the way you take the medicine doesn't work for you.

If you have trouble breathing, dizziness, or rashes, call your doctor right away. You may be having an allergic reaction to the pain medicine.

Don't Give up Hope. Your Pain Can Be Managed

If you are still having pain that is hard to control, you may want to talk with your health care team about seeing a pain or palliative care specialist. Whatever you do, don't give up. If one medicine doesn't work, there is almost always another one to try. Also, new medicines are created all the time. And unlike other medicines, there is no "right" dose for many pain medicines. Your dose may be more or less than someone else's. The right dose is the one that relieves your pain and makes you feel better.

5. MEDICINES TO TREAT CANCER PAIN

There Is More Than One Way to Treat Pain

Your doctor prescribes medicine based on the kind of pain you have and how severe it is. In studies, these medicines have been shown to help control cancer pain.

Doctors use three main groups of drugs for pain: nonopioids, opioids, and other types. You may also hear the term *analgesics* used for these pain relievers. Some are stronger than others. It helps to know the different kinds of medicines, why and how they're used, how you take them, and what side effects you might expect.

1. Nonopioids — For Mild to Moderate Pain

Nonopioids are drugs used to treat mild to moderate pain, fever, and swelling. On a scale of 0 to 10, a nonopioid may be used if you rate your pain from 1 to 4. These medicines are stronger than most people realize. In many cases, they are all you'll need to relieve your pain. You just need to be sure to take them regularly.

You can buy most nonopioids without a prescription. *But you still need to talk with your doctor before taking them.* Some of them may have things added to them that you need to know about. And they do have side effects. Common ones, such as nausea, itching, or drowsiness, usually go away after a few days. *Do not* take more than the label says unless your doctor tells you to do so.

Nonopioids include:

- *Acetaminophen, which you may know as Tylenol®*
  Acetaminophen reduces pain. It is not helpful with inflammation. Most of the time, people don't have side effects from a normal dose of acetaminophen. But taking large doses of this medicine every day for a long time can damage your liver. Drinking alcohol with the typical dose can also damage the liver.
  Make sure you tell the doctor that you're taking acetaminophen. Sometimes it is used in other pain medicines, so you may not realize that you're taking more than you should. Also, your doctor may not want you to take acetaminophen too often if you're getting chemotherapy. The medicine can cover up a fever, hiding the fact that you might have an infection.
- *Nonsteroidal anti-inflammatory drugs (NSAIDs), such as ibuprofen (which you may know as Advil® or Motrin®) and aspirin*
  NSAIDs help control pain and inflammation. With NSAIDs, the most common side effect is stomach upset or indigestion, especially in older people. Eating food or drinking milk when you take these drugs may stop this from happening.

NSAIDs may also keep blood from clotting the way it should. This means that it's harder to stop bleeding after you've hurt yourself. NSAIDs can also sometimes cause bleeding in the stomach.

Tell your doctor if:

- Your stools become darker than normal
- You notice bleeding from your rectum
- You have an upset stomach
- You have heartburn symptoms
- You cough up blood

Acetaminophen and NSAIDs at a Glance

Type	Other Names	Action	Side Effects
Acetaminophen	Tylenol®	Reduces pain and fever	Large doses can damage the liver. May cause liver damage if you drink three or more alcoholic drinks a day.
			Lowers fever. Talk to your doctor if your body temperature is above normal (98.6°) and you are taking this medicine.
NSAIDs (aspirin, ibuprofen, naproxen)		Reduces pain, inflammation (swelling), and fever	Can upset the stomach.
	Bayer® (aspirin)		Can cause bleeding of the stomach lining, especially if you drink alcohol (wine, beer, etc.).
	Ecotrin® (aspirin)		Can cause kidney problems, especially in the elderly or those with existing kidney problems.
	Advil® (ibuprofen) Motrin® (ibuprofen)		Can cause heart problems, especially in those who already have heart disease. However, aspirin does not cause heart problems.
	Nuprin® (ibuprofen)		Avoid these medicines if you are on anticancer drugs that may cause bleeding.
	Aleve® (naproxen)		Lowers fever. Talk to your doctor if your body temperature is above normal (98.6°) and you are taking this medicine.

What to Avoid When Taking NSAIDs

Some people have conditions that NSAIDs can make worse. In general, you should avoid these drugs if you:

- Are allergic to aspirin
- Are getting chemotherapy
- Are on steroid medicines
- Have stomach ulcers or a history of ulcers, gout, or bleeding disorders
- Are taking prescription medicines for arthritis
- Have kidney problems
- Have heart problems

- Are planning surgery within a week
- Are taking blood-thinning medicine (such as heparin or Coumadin®)

2. Opioids — For Moderate to Severe Pain

If you're having moderate to severe pain, your doctor may recommend that you take stronger drugs called opioids. Opioids are sometimes called narcotics. You must have a doctor's prescription to take them. They are often taken with aspirin, ibuprofen, and acetaminophen.

Common opioids include:

- Codeine
- Fentanyl
- Hydromorphone (e.g., Dilaudid®)
- Levorphanol
- Meperidine (e.g., Demerol®)
- Methadone
- Morphine
- Oxycodone (e.g., OxyContin®)
- Oxymorphone

Getting Relief with Opioids

Over time, people who take opioids for pain sometimes find that they need to take larger doses to get relief. This is caused by more pain, the cancer getting worse, or medicine *tolerance*. When a medicine doesn't give you enough pain relief, your doctor may increase the dose and how often you take it. He or she can also prescribe a stronger drug. Both methods are safe and effective under your doctor's care. *Do not increase the dose of medicine on your own.*

Managing and Preventing Side Effects

Some pain medicines may cause:

- Constipation (trouble passing stools)
- Drowsiness (feeling sleepy)
- Nausea (upset stomach)
- Vomiting (throwing up)

Side effects vary with each person. It's important to talk to your doctor often about any side effects you're having. If needed, he or she can change your medicines or the doses you're taking. They can also add other medicines to your pain control plan to help your side effects.

Keep in mind that constipation will only go away if it's treated. But don't let any side effects stop you from getting your pain controlled. Your health care team can talk with you about other ways to relieve them. There are solutions to getting your pain under control.

Other less common side effects include:

- Dizziness
- Confusion
- Breathing problems
- Itching
- Trouble urinating

Constipation

Almost everyone taking opioids has some constipation. This happens because opioids cause the stool to move more slowly through your system, so your body takes more time to absorb water from the stool. The stool then becomes hard.

You can control or prevent constipation by taking these steps:

- Ask your doctor about giving you *laxatives* and *stool softeners* when you first start taking opioids. Taking these right when you start taking pain medicine may prevent the problem.
- Drink plenty of liquids. Drinking 8 to 10 glasses of liquid each day will help keep stools soft.
- Eat foods high in fiber, including raw fruits with the skin left on, vegetables, and whole grain breads and cereals.
- Exercise as much as you are able. Any movement, such as light walking, will help.
- Call your doctor if you have not had a bowel movement in 2 days or more.

Drowsiness

Some opioids cause drowsiness. Or, if your pain has kept you from sleeping, you may sleep more at first when you begin taking opioids. The drowsiness could go away after a few days.

If you're are tired or drowsy:

- Don't walk up and down stairs alone.
- Don't do anything where you need to be alert—driving, using machines or equipment, or anything else that requires focus.

Call your doctor if the drowsiness is severe or doesn't go away after a few days.

- You may have to take a smaller dose more often or change medicines.
- It may be that the medicine isn't relieving your pain, and the pain is keeping you awake at night.
- Your other medicines may be causing the drowsiness.
- Your doctor may decide to add a new drug that will help you stay awake.

Nausea and Vomiting

Nausea and vomiting could go away after a few days of taking opioids. However, if your nausea or vomiting prevents you from taking your medicine, call your doctor right away. You should also call if any breathing problems develop.

These tips may help:

- Stay in bed for an hour or so after taking your medicine if you feel sick when walking around. This kind of nausea is like feeling seasick. Some over-the-counter drugs may help, too. But be sure to check with your doctor before taking any other medicines.
- Your doctor may want to change or add medicines, or prescribe antinausea drugs.
- Ask your doctor if something else could be making you feel sick. It might be related to your cancer or another medicine you're taking. Constipation can also add to nausea.

Starting a New Pain Medicine

Some pain medicines can make you feel sleepy when you first take them. This usually goes away within a few days. Also, some people get dizzy or feel confused. Tell your doctor if any of these symptoms persist. Changing your dose or the type of medicine can usually solve the problem.

What to Watch out for When Taking Pain Medicine

All drugs must be taken carefully. Here are a few things to remember when you are taking opioids:

- *Take your medicines as directed.* Also, don't split, chew, or crush them, unless suggested by your doctor.
- *Doctors will adjust the pain medicine dose so that you get the right amount for your body.* That's why it's important that only one doctor prescribes your opioids. Make sure that you bring your list of medicines to each visit. That way, your health care team is aware of your pain control plan.
- *Combining pain medicine with alcohol or tranquilizers can be dangerous.* You could have trouble breathing or feel confused, anxious, or dizzy.

Tell your doctor how much and how often you:

- Drink alcohol
- Take tranquilizers, sleeping pills, or *antidepressants*
- Take any other medicines that make you sleepy

How to Stop Taking Opioids

You may be able to take less medicine when the pain gets better. You may even be able to stop taking opioids. But it's important to stop taking opioids slowly, with your doctor's advice. When pain medicines are taken for long periods of time, your body gets used to them. If the medicines are stopped or suddenly reduced, a condition called *withdrawal* may occur. This is why the doses should be lowered slowly. This has *no* relation to being addicted.

Stopping your pain medicines slowly prevents withdrawal symptoms. But if you stop taking opioids suddenly, you may start feeling like you have the flu. You may sweat and have diarrhea or other symptoms. If this happens, tell your doctor or nurse. He or she can treat these symptoms, which usually resolve quickly.

3. Other Types of Pain Medicine
Doctors also prescribe other types of medicine to relieve cancer pain. They can be used along with nonopioids and opioids. Some include:

- **Antidepressants**: Some drugs can be used for more than one purpose. For example, antidepressants are used to treat depression, but they may also help relieve tingling and burning pain. Nerve damage from radiation, surgery, or chemotherapy can cause this type of pain.
- **Antiseizure medicines (anticonvulsants)**: Like antidepressants, anticonvulsants or antiseizure drugs can also be used to help control tingling or burning from nerve injury.
- **Steroids**: Steroids are mainly used to treat pain caused by swelling.

Be sure to ask your health care team about the common side effects of these medicines.

How Medicine Is Given
To relieve cancer pain, doctors often prescribe pills or liquids. But there are also other ways to take medicines, such as:

- **Mouth**: Some pain medicine can be put inside the cheek or under the tongue.
- **Injections (shots)**: There are two different kinds of shots:
  - **Under the skin**: Medicine is placed just under the skin using a small needle. These are called *subcutaneous* injections.
  - **In the vein**: Medicine goes directly into the vein through a needle. These are called *intravenous (IV)* injections. *Patient-controlled analgesia (PCA)* pumps are often used with these kinds of injections. PCA pumps let you push a button to give yourself a dose of pain medicine.
- **Skin patches**: These bandage-like patches go on the skin. They slowly but steadily, release medicine.
- **Rectal suppositories**: These are capsules or pills that you put inside your rectum. The medicine dissolves and is absorbed by the body.
- **In or around the spinal cord**: Medicine is placed between the wall of the spinal canal and the covering of the spinal cord.

Questions to Ask Your Health Care Team About Your Pain Medicine

- How much medicine should I take? How often?
- If my pain doesn't go away, can I take more medicine? How much should I increase the dose?
- Should I call you before taking more medicine?
- How long does the medicine last?
- What if I forget to take my medicine or take it later than I was supposed to?
- Should I take my medicine with food?
- How much liquid should I drink with the medicine?
- How long does it take for the medicine to start working? Is it safe to drink alcohol (wine, beer, etc.), drive, or run machinery after I've taken the medicine?
- What other medicines can I take with the pain medicine?
- What are the side effects? How can I prevent them?
- What should I call you about right away?

Other Ways to Relieve Pain

Medicine doesn't always relieve pain in some people. In these cases, doctors use other treatments to reduce pain:

- **Radiation therapy**: Different forms of radiation energy are used to shrink the tumor and reduce pain. Often one treatment is enough to help with the pain. But sometimes several treatments are needed.
- **Neurosurgery**: A surgeon cuts the nerves that carry pain messages to your brain.
- **Nerve blocks**: Anesthesiologists inject pain medicine into or around the nerve or into the spine to relieve pain.
- **Surgery**: A surgeon removes all or part of a tumor to relieve pain. This is especially helpful when a tumor presses on nerves or other parts of the body.
- **Chemotherapy**: Anticancer drugs are used to reduce the size of a tumor, which may help with the pain.

- **Transcutaneous Electric Nerve Stimulation (TENS)**: TENS uses a gentle electric current to relieve pain. The current comes from a small power pack that you can hold or attach to yourself.

Your Pharmacist

Your Pharmacist is an important member of your health care team. He or she can answer many questions about your medicines, such as how to take them, or what side effects they have. It's a pharmacist's job to stay up-to-date and informed about cancer drugs.

If possible, try to use just one pharmacy. This way, all your prescriptions will be on file in one system. Some pharmacies even have systems that give warnings if newly ordered medicines could interact or interfere with others that someone is already taking.

6. MEDICINE TOLERANCE AND ADDICTION

When Treating Cancer Pain, Addiction Is Rarely a Problem

Addiction is when people can't control their seeking or craving for something. They continue to take medicine or do something even when it causes them harm. Often people are taking medicines when they do not have pain. They take it for psychological reasons, not physical. But people with cancer need strong medicine to help control their pain. Yet some people are so afraid of becoming addicted to pain medicine that they won't take it. Family members may also worry that their loved ones will get addicted to pain medicine. Therefore, they sometimes encourage loved ones to "hold off" between doses But even though they may mean well, it's best to take your medicine as prescribed.

People in pain get the most relief when they take their medicines on schedule. And don't be afraid to ask for larger doses if you need them. As mentioned earlier, developing a tolerance to pain medicine is common. But taking cancer pain medicine is not likely to cause addiction. If you're not a drug addict, you won't become one. Even if you have had an addiction problem before, you still deserve good pain management. Talk with your doctor or nurse about your concerns.

"If you're worried about addiction, ask yourself one question. If you didn't have this pain, would you want this medicine? The answer is usually no." — Robin

Tolerance to Pain Medicine Sometimes Happens

Some people think that they have to save stronger medicines for later. They're afraid that their bodies will get used to the medicine and that it won't work anymore. But medicine doesn't stop working—it just doesn't work as well as it once did. As you keep taking a medicine over time, you may need a change in your pain control plan to get the same amount of relief.

This is called *tolerance*. Tolerance is a common issue in cancer pain treatment.

Medicine Tolerance Is Not the Same As Addiction

As mentioned, medicine tolerance happens when your body gets used to the medicine you're taking. Each person's body is different. Many people don't develop a tolerance to opioids. But if tolerance happens to you, don't worry.

Under your doctor's care, you can:

- Increase your dose
- Add a new kind of medicine
- Change the kind of medicine that you're taking for pain

The goal is to relieve your pain. Increasing the dose to overcome tolerance does not lead to addiction.

Taking Pain Medicine Will Not Cause You to "Get High"

Most people do not "get high" or lose control when they take cancer pain medicines as prescribed by the doctor. Some pain medicines can cause you to feel sleepy when you first take them. This feeling usually goes away within a few days. On occasion, people get dizzy or feel confused when they take pain medicines. Tell your doctor or nurse if this happens to you. Changing your dose or type of medicine can usually solve this problem.

7. OTHER WAYS TO CONTROL PAIN

Along with your pain medicine, your health care team may suggest you try other methods to control your pain. However, unlike pain medicine, some of these methods have not been tested in cancer pain studies. But they may help improve your quality of life by helping you with your pain, as well as stress, anxiety, and coping with cancer. Some of these methods are called complementary or integrative.

These treatments include everything from cold packs, massage, acupuncture, hypnosis, and imagery to biofeedback, meditation, and therapeutic touch. Once you learn how, you can do some of them by yourself. For others, you may have to see a specialist to receive these treatments. If you do, ask if they are licensed experts.

Acupuncture

Acupuncture is a form of Chinese medicine. It involves inserting very thin, metal needles into the skin at certain points of the body. *(Applying pressure to these points with just the thumbs or fingertips is called acupressure.)* The goal is to change the body's energy flow so it can heal itself.

When receiving this treatment, you may have a slight ache, dull pain, tingling, or electrical-feeling sensation for a few seconds after the needles are inserted. Once the needles are in place, though, you shouldn't feel any discomfort. They remain in place for 15 to 30 minutes. However, it may be more or less, depending on what the practitioner suggests.

Acupuncture has been shown to help with nausea and vomiting related to cancer treatment. And some studies have shown it may help with cancer pain. Before getting acupuncture, talk with your health care team to make sure it's safe for your type of cancer. If it is, your health care team can suggest a licensed acupuncturist. Many hospitals and cancer centers have one on staff.

Biofeedback

Biofeedback uses machines to teach you how to control certain body functions, such as heart rate, breathing, and muscle tension. You probably never think of these body functions because they happen on their own. But learning how to control them may help you relax and cope with pain. Biofeedback is often used with other pain relief methods. If you're interested in trying this method, you must see a licensed biofeedback technician.

Distraction

Distraction is simply turning your focus to something other than the pain. It may be used alone to manage mild pain, or used with medicines to help with acute pain, such as pain related to procedures or tests. Or you may try it while waiting for your pain medicine to start working.

More than likely, you've done this method without realizing it. For example, watching television and listening to music are good ways to distract your mind. In fact, any activity that can focus your attention can be used for distraction. You can count, sing, or pray. You could try slow rhythmic breathing or repeat certain phrases over and over again, such as "I can cope."

You could do certain activities that take your mind from the pain. Some of these may be crafts or hobbies, reading, going to a movie, or visiting friends.

Heat and Cold

Heat may relieve sore muscles, while cold may numb the pain. However, ask your doctor if it is safe to use either during treatment. Do not use them for more than 10 minutes at a time. And *do not* use heat or cold over any area where circulation is poor.

For cold, try plastic gel packs that remain soft even when frozen. You can find them in drug and medical-supply stores. Of course, you always can use ice cubes wrapped in a towel or frozen water in a paper cup.

For heat, you can use a heating pad. But you also can try gel packs heated in hot water, hot-water bottles, a hot, moist towel, and hot baths and showers. Be careful not to leave heat on too long to avoid burns.

Hypnosis

Hypnosis is a trance-like state of relaxed and focused attention. People describe it as a lot like the way they feel when they first wake up in the morning. Their eyes are closed, but they're aware of what's going on around them. In this relaxed state, people's minds are usually more receptive or open to suggestion. As a result, hypnosis can be used to block the awareness of pain or to help you change the sensation of pain to a more pleasant one.

You'll need to see a person who is trained in hypnosis, often a psychologist or psychiatrist. He or she may also be able to teach you how to place yourself in a trance-like state, by making positive suggestions to yourself.

Imagery

Imagery is like a daydream. You close your eyes and create images in your mind to help you relax, feel less anxious, and sleep. You daydream using all of your senses – sight, touch, hearing, smell, and taste. For example, you may want to think of a place or activity that made you happy in the past. You could explore this scene, which could help reduce your pain both during and after you try it.

If you have to stay in bed or can't leave the house, imagery may help. It may lessen the closed-in feelings you have after being indoors for a long time.

Massage

Massage may help reduce pain and anxiety. It may also help with fatigue and stress. It is pressing, rubbing, and kneading parts of the body with hands or special tools. For pain, a steady, circular motion near the pain site may work best. Massage may also help relieve tension and increase blood flow. Deep or intense pressure should not be used with cancer patients unless their healthcare team says it's okay to do so.

Meditation

Meditation is a form of mind-body medicine used to help relax the body and quiet the mind. It may help with pain, as well as with worry, stress, or depression.

People who are meditating use certain techniques such as focusing attention on something, like a word or phrase, an object, or the breath. They may sit, lie down, walk, or be in any other position that makes them feel comfortable. A goal while meditating is to try to have an open attitude toward distracting thoughts or emotions. When they occur, attention is gently brought back to breathing or the silent repeating of phrases.

> "I began meditating as a way to help relieve my pain and calm myself. I can't avoid medicine, but I feel like I don't have to take as much." — Anna

Relaxation

Relaxation reduces pain or keeps it from getting worse by getting rid of tension in your muscles. It may help you sleep and give you more energy. Relaxation may also reduce anxiety and help you cope with stress.

The most common methods of relaxation are:

- **Visual concentration**: When you stare at an object.
- **Breathing and muscle tensing**: This is breathing in and tensing the muscles, then breathing out while letting your muscles go. See "Relaxation Exercises" later in this chapter for an exercise on how to use breathing and muscle tensing.
- **Slow rhythmic breathing**: To do this, you breathe slowly in and out while concentrating on an object. You can add imagery to slow rhythmic breathing or listen to music too. See "Relaxation Exercises" later in this chapter for an exercise on how to use slow rhythmic breathing.

Sometimes, relaxation is hard if you're in severe pain. You could try using some of the methods that are quick and easy. These may be rhythmic massage or breathing and muscle tensing. Some people use music or other types of art therapy to help them relax.

Sometimes breathing too deeply can cause shortness of breath. If this happens, take shallow breaths or breathe more slowly. Also, as you start to relax, you may fall asleep. If you don't want to sleep, sit in a hard chair or set a timer or alarm before you start the exercise.

Other Methods

Here are some other ways people have tried to find relief from cancer pain.

- **Physical Therapy**: Exercises or methods used to help restore strength, increase movement to muscles, and relieve pain.
- **Reiki**: A form of energy medicine in which the provider places his or her hands on or near the patient. The intent is to transmit what is believed to be a life force energy called qi (or chi).
- **Tai Chi**: A mind-body practice that is a series of slow, gentle movements with a focus on breathing and concentration. The thought is that it helps what is believed to be a life force energy (called qi) flow through the body.
- **Yoga**: Systems of stretches and poses with special focus given to breathing. It is meant to calm the nervous system and balance the body, mind, and spirit. There are different types of yoga, so ask about which ones would be best for you.

Make sure that you see a licensed expert when trying physical therapy, massage, hypnosis, or acupuncture.

To learn more about complementary treatments for pain:

- Talk with your doctor, nurse, or oncology social worker.
- See the NCI chapter *Thinking About Complementary & Alternative Medicine: A Guide for People With Cancer.*
- Contact the National Center for Complementary and Alternative Medicine at 1-888-644-6226 or online at http://nccam.nih.gov.
- See the web site for the NCI Office of Cancer Complementary and Alternative Medicine at http://www.cancer

Remember: Always talk with your doctor before using any complementary pain treatments. Some may interfere with your cancer treatment.

8. YOUR FEELINGS AND PAIN

Having pain and cancer affects every part of your life.

It can affect not only your body, but your thoughts and feelings as well. Whether you have a lot of pain or a little, if it's constant, you may feel like you aren't able to focus on anything else. It may keep you from doing things and seeing people that you normally do. This can be upsetting and may feel like a cycle that never seems to end.

Sometimes things that people used to take for granted aren't as easy anymore. These may include cooking, getting dressed, or just moving around. Some people can't work because of the pain or have to cut back on their hours. They may worry about money. Limits on work and everyday life may also make people less social, wanting to see others less often.

Research shows that people in pain may feel sad or anxious and may get depressed more often. At other times they may feel irritable, or angry and frustrated. And they can feel lonely, even if they have others around them.

A common result of having cancer and being in pain is fear. For many, pain and fear together feel like suffering. People get upset worrying about the future. They focus their thoughts on things that may or may not happen. You may feel fear about many things, such as fear of:

- The cancer getting worse
- The pain being too much to handle
- Your job or daily tasks becoming too hard to do
- Not being able to attend special trips or events
- Loss of control

This rollercoaster of feelings often makes people look for the meaning that cancer and pain have in their life. Some question why this could happen to them. They wonder what they did to deserve it. Others may turn to religion or explore their spirituality more, asking for guidance and strength.

Don't Lose Hope

If you have feelings like these, know that you're not alone. Many people with cancer pain have had these kinds of feelings. Having negative thoughts is normal. And some people have positive thoughts, too, finding benefits in facing cancer. But if your negative thoughts overwhelm you, don't ignore your feelings. Help is there for you if you're distressed or unsure about your future.

Finding Support

There are many people who can help you. You can talk with oncology social workers, health psychologists, or other mental health experts at your hospital or clinic.

Your health care team can help you find a counselor who is trained to help people with long-term illnesses. These people can help you talk about what you are going through and find answers to your concerns. They may suggest medicine that will help you feel better if you need it.

Many people say that they regain a sense of control and well-being after talking with people in their spiritual or religious community. A leader from one of these groups may be able to offer support, too. Many are trained to help people cope with illness.

Also, many hospitals have a staff chaplain who can counsel people of all faiths.

You can also talk with friends or others in your community. Some join a support group. Cancer support groups are made up of people who share their feelings about coping with cancer. They can meet in person, by phone, or over the Internet. They may help you gain new insights and ideas on how to cope. To find a support group for you, talk with your doctor, nurse, or oncology social worker.

> "I can't help Feeling Frustrated with all that's going on in my liFe. Between my cancer treatments and the pain, I get upset and angry. Sometimes I really need someone to talk to— someone who understands what I'm going through." — Carlos

How Your Pain Affects Your Loved Ones

Chronic or severe pain affects everyone who loves and takes care of you. It can be hard for family members and friends to watch someone close to them be in pain.

Like you, your loved ones may feel angry, anxious, and lonely. They may feel helpless because they can't make you feel better. They may even feel guilty that you have pain while they don't. Or they may feel loss, because your pain keeps you from doing things you like to do.

It's natural for family members and friends to have these emotions. It may help if everyone understands that these emotions exist and that no one needs to face them alone.

Let your family members know it's okay for them to get help. Like you, they can talk to a counselor or join a support group. Encourage them to ask the oncology social worker about the options that are available for them.

Talking with Family Members

You may want to let family members and friends know how you're feeling. For some, this can be hard or awkward. Some people say that they want to avoid upsetting those closest to them. Others say that they don't want to seem negative. But open and honest communication can help everyone. Letting others know about your pain may help them understand what you are going through. They can then look for ways to help you. Your loved ones may also feel better knowing that they're helping to make you feel more comfortable.

Family Problems before Your Cancer

Any problems your family had before you got cancer are likely to be more intense now. Or maybe your family just doesn't communicate very well. If this is the case, you can ask a social worker to set up a family meeting for you. During these meetings, the doctor can explain treatment goals and issues. And you and your family members can state your wishes for care. These meetings can also give everyone a chance to express their feelings in the open. Remember, there are many people you can turn to at this time.

9. Financial Issues

"My doctor told me about a pain control technique that he thought would help me. I was a little worried about how I would pay For it. It took one phone call to my insurance company, and my questions were answered." — Terry

When you're in pain, the last thing you want to think about is paying for your medicine. Yet money worries have stopped many people from getting the pain treatment they need. Talk with your oncology social worker if you have questions. He or she should be able to direct you to resources in your area. Here are some general tips:

Insurance

When dealing with health insurance, you might want to:

- Call your insurance company and find out what treatments are covered. Sometimes insurance companies pay for only certain types of medicines. If the medicine you need isn't covered, your doctor may need to write a special appeal letter. Or your doctor may need to prescribe a different treatment.
- Ask if your insurance company can give you a case manager to help you with your coverage.
- Check to make sure that your plan will cover any specialists your doctor refers you to. If it does not, check with your insurance company to see which doctors are included in your plan. Ask your doctor to refer you to someone on your plan's list.
- Find out whether you have to pay copayments up front and how much they cost.
- Find out how you should pay your balance. For example, do you file a claim? Does the insurance company pay first? Or do you pay and get reimbursed?
- Tell the insurance company if you believe you've received an incorrect bill. You should also tell your doctor or the hospital or clinic that sent the bill. Don't be afraid to ask questions.

Government Health Insurance Medicare

Medicare is health insurance for people age 65 or older. However, people under 65 who are on kidney dialysis or have certain disabilities may also qualify.

Medicare Part B only pays for outpatient medicine given by a pump or by vein. It doesn't pay for pills, patches, or liquids.

Medicare Part D is a benefit that covers outpatient prescription medicines. It comes from private insurance plans that have a contract with Medicare. These plans vary in what they cost and the medicines they cover. Find out which medicines a plan covers before you join to make sure that it meets your needs. You should also know how much your copays and *deductible* will be.

Medicaid

Medicaid gives health benefits to low income people and their families. Some may have no health insurance or not enough, and therefore need this help.

If you have Medicaid, you should know that it pays for medicine given by mouth (*orally*) or by vein (intravenous). Each state has its own rules about who is eligible for Medicaid.

> To learn more about Medicare and Medicaid talk with your oncology social worker. You can also go to the Medicare and Medicaid Web site, www.cms.hhs.gov, or call the helpline at 1-800-MEDICARE (1-800-633-4227). Specialists can answer your questions or direct you to free counseling in your area.

Other Advice

Don't be embarrassed to tell your health care team if you're having trouble paying for your medicine. They may be able to prescribe other medicine that better fits your budget.

If you feel that you're overwhelmed, the stress may seem like too much to handle. You might try getting help with financial planning. Talk with the business office where you get treatment. There are many free consumer credit counseling agencies and groups. Talk with your oncology social worker about your choices. You can also contact the NCI's Cancer Information Service (CIS) and ask for help. They have a database, *National Organizations that Offer Cancer-Related Services,* that may help you. See the Resources section later in this chapter for ways to contact NCI.

Tips for Saving Money on Pain Medicine

If the cost of pain medicine is an issue for you, consider the following tips:

- Ask your doctor if there are *generic* brands of your medicine available. These usually cost less than brand-name medicines.
- Ask your doctor for medicine samples before paying for a prescription. You can't get samples of opioids. But you can ask your doctor to write only part of the prescription. This way you can make sure that the medicine works for you before buying the rest of it. This will only help if you pay by the amount you buy. For some insurance plans, you pay the same amount for part of or the whole prescription. Find out what will work best for you.
- Ask about drug companies that have special programs to give free drugs to patients in financial need. Your doctor should know about these programs.
- Remember that pills may cost less than other forms of medicine.
- Use a bulk-order mail pharmacy. But first make sure that the medicine works for you. Also, be aware that you can't order opioids in bulk or through the mail. Ask your oncology social worker or pharmacist about bulk-order mail pharmacies.
- Contact NeedyMeds.
  They are a nonprofit organization that helps people who cannot afford medicine or health care costs. Go to http://www.needymeds.com, or ask someone to do it for you.

REFLECTION

You can take control of your pain. Work with your doctor and the other members of your health care team to find the best plan for you. Read the tips in this chapter and make them work for you. Don't lose hope. You don't have to accept pain as a normal part of cancer or treatment. You deserve to have the best care and support there is.

RESOURCES

You can get information about cancer from many sources. Some are listed here. You may also want to check for more information from support groups in your community.

Federal Agencies

- **National Cancer Institute**

Offers comprehensive research-based information for patients, families, health professionals, and the general public. Topics include cancer prevention, screening, diagnosis, treatment, genetics, and supportive care. NCI's web site lists clinical trials and specific cancer topics in NCI's Physician Data Query (PDQ) database.

Toll-free: 1-800-4-CANCER (1-800-422-6237)
Online: http://www.cancer or http://www.cancer.gov/espanol
Chat online: LiveHelp, NCI's instant messaging service, at http://www.cancer
E-mail: cancergovstaff@mail.nih.gov
Publications: Order online at http://www.cancer or call 1-800-4-CANCER (1-800-422-6237)

- **Centers for Medicare & Medicaid Services (CMS)**

Has information about patient rights, prescription drugs, and health insurance issues, including Medicare and Medicaid.

Toll-free: 1-800-MEDICARE (1-800-633-4227)
Online: http://www.medicare.gov (for Medicare information) or http://www.cms.hhs.gov (for other information)

- **National Center for Complementary and Alternative Medicine (NCCAM)**

Part of the National Institutes of Health. It funds and studies medical practices that are not commonly used as standard care. It rates how well these different practices work and shares this information with the public.
Toll-free: 1-888-644-6226
TTY: 1-888-644-6226
Online: http://nccam.nih.gov

Private/Nonprofit Organizations

- **American Cancer Society (ACS)**

Mission is to end cancer as a major health problem through prevention, saving lives, and relieving suffering. ACS works toward these goals through research, education, advocacy, and service. The organization's National Cancer Information Center answers questions 24 hours a day, 7 days a week.
Toll-free: 1-800-ACS-2345 (1-800-227-2345)
TTY: 1-866-228-4327
Online: http://www.cancer

- **American Pain Foundation**

Serves people with pain through information, advocacy, and support; pain and resource information, practical help and publications are available through toll-free telephone service and website.
Toll-free: 1-888-615-PAIN (1-888-615-7246)
Online: http://www.painfoundation.org

- **CancerCare**

Offers free support, information, and financial and practical help to people with cancer and their loved ones.
Toll-free: 1-800-813-HOPE (1-800-813-4673)
Online: http://www.cancercare.org

- **Cancer Support Community**

Cancer Support Community is a national organization that provides support groups, stress reduction and cancer education workshops, nutrition guidance, exercise sessions, and social events.

Phone: 1-888-793-WELL (1-888-793-9355)
Web site: http://www.cancersupportcommunity.org

- **Center to Advance Palliative Care**

Goal is to increase the availability of quality palliative care services for people facing serious illness. Offers training and assistance to health care professionals.
Phone: 1-212-201-2670
Online: http://www.capc.org
For patients and families: http://www.getpalliativecare.org

- **National Coalition for Cancer Survivorship (NCCS)**

Gives out information on cancer support, employment, financial and legal issues, advocacy, and related issues.
Toll-free: 1-877-NCCS-YES (1-877-622-7937)
Online: http://www.canceradvocacy.org

- **National Hospice and Palliative Care Organization (NHPCO)**

Has information on hospice care, local hospice programs, advance directives in different states, and finding a local health care provider. It offers education and materials on palliative and end-of-life issues through its Caring Connections program, as well as links to other organizations and resources.
Toll-free: 1-800-658-8898
Online: http://www.nhpco.org

- **Caring Connections**

Toll-free: 1-800-658-8898
Online: http://www.caringinfo.org

- **NeedyMeds**

Lists medicine assistance programs available from drug companies. NOTE: Usually patients cannot apply directly to these programs. Ask your doctor, nurse, or social worker to contact them.
Online: http://www.needymeds.com

- **Patient Advocate Foundation**

Offers education, legal counseling, and referrals concerning managed care, insurance, financial issues, job discrimination, and debt crisis matters.

Toll-free: 1-800-532-5274
Online: http://www.patientadvocate.org

PAIN CONTROL RECORD

You can use a chart like this to keep a record of how well your medicine is working. Some people call it a pain diary. Describe the amount of pain you feel using the way that works best for you. You can use words, numbers on a scale from 0 to 10, or even draw a face. Take the chart with you when you visit your doctor.

Date	Time	Describe the pain you feel	Pain level	Action taken
6/8 (example)	8am	stabbing pain in side	9	
6/10 (example)	all day	dull ache in legs	5	

Medicines You Are Taking Now

You can make a form to record all medicines—not just pain medicines—that you are taking. This information will help your doctor keep track of all your medicines.

Date	Medicine	Dose	How often taken	How well is it working?	Prescribing doctor

Pain Medicines You Have Taken in the Past

You can make a form to record the pain medicines you have taken in the past. It will help your doctor understand what has and hasn't worked.

Date	Medicine	Dose	How often taken	Side effects	Reason for stopping

HOW TO USE IMAGERY

Imagery usually works best with your eyes closed. To begin, create an image in your mind. For example, you may want to think of a place or activity that made you happy in the past. Explore this place or activity. Notice how calm you feel.

If you have severe pain, you may imagine yourself as a person without pain. In your image, cut the wires that send pain signals from one part of your body to another. Or you may want to imagine a ball of healing energy. Others have found this exercise to be very helpful:

- Close your eyes and breathe slowly. As you breathe in, say silently and slowly to yourself, "In, one, two,' and as you breathe out, say "Out, one, two.' Do this for a few minutes.
- Imagine a ball of healing energy forming in your lungs or on your chest. Imagine it forming and taking shape.
- When you're ready, imagine that the air you breathe in blows this ball of energy to the area where you feel pain. Once there, the ball heals and relaxes you. You may imagine that the ball gets bigger and bigger as it takes away more of your discomfort.
- When you breathe out, imagine the air blowing the ball away from your body. As it goes, all your pain goes with it.
- Repeat the last two steps each time you breathe in and out.
- To end the imagery, count slowly to three, breathe in deeply, open your eyes, and say silently to yourself, "I feel alert and relaxed.'

Relaxation Exercises

You may relax either sitting up or lying down, preferably in a quiet place. Make sure you're comfortable. Don't cross your arms or legs because you could cut off circulation. If you're lying down, you may want to put a small pillow under your neck and knees.

Once you're comfortable and your eyes are closed, you could try any of the following relaxation methods:

Breathing and Muscle Tensing
- Breathe in deeply.

- At the same time, tense your muscles or group of muscles. For example, you can squeeze your eyes shut, frown, or clench your teeth. Or, you could make a fist, stiffen your arms and legs, or draw your legs and arms up into a ball and hold as tightly as you can.
- Hold your breath and keep your muscles tense for a second or two.
- Let go. Breathe out and let your body go limp.

Slow Rhythmic Breathing

- Stare at an object or shut your eyes and think of a peaceful scene. Take a slow, deep breath.
- As you breathe in, tense your muscles. As you breathe out, relax your muscles and feel the tension leaving.
- Remain relaxed and begin breathing slowly and comfortably, taking about nine or 12 breaths a minute. To maintain a slow, even rhythm, you can silently say to yourself, "in, one, two; out, one, two."
- If you ever feel out of breath, take a deep breath, and continue the slow breathing.
- Each time you breathe out, feel yourself relaxing and going limp. Continue the slow, rhythmic breathing for up to 10 minutes, if you need it.
- To end the session, count silently and slowly from one to three. Open your eyes. Say to yourself, "I feel alert and relaxed." Begin moving slowly.

If you decide to use slow rhythmic breathing as a way to relax and reduce pain, you may want to try these tips. They can add to the experience.

- Listen to slow, familiar music through earphones.
- Once you're breathing slowly, slowly relax different parts of your body, one after the other. Start with your feet and work up to your head.
- Each time you breathe out, you can focus on a particular area of the body and feel it relaxing. Try to imagine the tension draining from the area.
- Consider using relaxation tapes. They often include each step on how to relax.

WORDS TO KNOW

Acupuncture (ACK-yu-punk-chur): Small needles are inserted into the skin at certain points of the body to relieve pain.

Acute pain: Pain that is very bad but lasts a fairly short time.

Addiction: (uh-DIK-shin): Drug craving, seeking, and use that you can't control.

Analgesic: A drug that reduces pain.

Anesthesiologist (an-uh-steez-ee-YAH-luh-jist): A doctor who specializes in giving medicines or other drugs that prevent or relieve pain.

Anticonvulsant (an-tee-kuhn-VUHL-sint): Medicine used to treat seizures that can also be used to control burning, stabbing, and tingling pain.

Antidepressant (an-tee-duh-PRES-int): Medicine used to treat depression that can also be used to relieve tingling, stabbing, or burning pain from damaged nerves.

Biofeedback: A way of learning to control some body functions such as heartbeat, blood pressure, and muscle tension with the help of special machines. This method may help control pain.

Breakthrough pain: An intense rise in pain that occurs suddenly or is felt for a short time. It can occur by itself or in relation to a certain activity. It may happen several times a day, even when you're taking the right dose of medicine.

Chemotherapy (kee-moh-THAIR-uh-pee): Treatment with anticancer medicines.

Chronic (KRAH-nik) **pain**: Pain that can range from mild to severe and is present for a long time.

Complementary treatment: Treatment used along with standard medical care.

Deductible: The amount you must pay for health care before insurance begins to pay.

Distraction: A pain relief method that takes the attention away from the pain.

Dose: The amount of medicine taken.

Generic: The scientific name of a drug, as opposed to the brand name. Also, drugs not protected by trademark.

Hypnosis (hip-NOH-sis): A person enters into a trance-like state, becomes more aware and focused, and is more open to suggestion.

Imagery: People think of pleasant images or scenes, such as waves hitting a beach, to help them relax.

Integrative medicine: Combines standard medical care and complementary and alternative medicine, for which there is some high-quality evidence of safety and effectiveness.

Intravenous (in-tra-VEE-nus): Within a blood vessel. Also called *IV*.

Intravenous infusion: A way of giving pain medicine into a vein or under the skin. An infusion flows in by gravity or a mechanical pump. It is different from an injection, which is pushed in by a syringe.

Laxative: Something you take to help you pass solid waste, or stool, from your body. There are many different kinds of laxatives.

Narcotics (nahr-KAH-tiks): See opioids.

Nerve block: Pain medicine is injected directly into or around a nerve or into the spine to block pain.

Neurologist: A doctor who specializes in the treatment of nervous system disorders.

Neuropathic (noor-AH-path-ik) **pain**: Pain that occurs when treatment damages the nerves.

Nonopioids (nahn-OH-pee-yoidz): Acetaminophen and nonsteroidal anti-inflammatory drugs (NSAIDs), such as aspirin, ibuprofen, and naproxen.

Nonprescription: Over-the-counter drugs that you can buy without a doctor's order.

NSAIDs (Nonsteroidal anti-inflammatory drugs): Medicines that control mild to moderate pain and inflammation and reduce fever. Can be used either alone or together with other medicines.

Oncologist (ahn-KAH-luh-jist): A doctor who specializes in the treatment of cancer.

Oncology (ahn-KAH-luh-jee): The study and treatment of cancer.

Onset of action: The length of time it takes for a medicine to start to work.

Opioids (OH-pee-yoidz): Also known as narcotics. They are used to treat moderate to severe pain. A prescription is needed for these medicines.

Oral: By mouth.

Pain threshold: The point at which a person becomes aware of pain.

Palliative (PAL-ee-yuh-tiv) **care**: Care given to improve quality of life and/or slow cancer's growth. The goal is to prevent or treat the symptoms, side effects, and psychological and emotional problems of the disease. Not meant to be a cure.

Patient-controlled analgesia (an-ull-JEEZ-ya) **(PCA)**: A way for a person with pain to control the amount of pain medicine he or she receives. When pain relief is needed, the person can press a button on a computerized pump connected to a small tube inserted into the vein or under the skin. Pushing the button delivers a preset dose of pain medicine.

Phantom pain: When pain or other unpleasant feelings are felt from a missing (phantom) body part that has been removed by surgery.

Physical therapy: Treatment for pain in muscles, nerves, joints, and bones. This treatment uses exercise, electrical stimulation, and hydrotherapy, as well as massage, heat, cold, and electrical devices.

Prescription: A doctor's order.

Qi (chee): What is believed to be a life force energy.

Radiation therapy: Treatment with high-energy x-rays to kill or control cancer cells. **Relaxation techniques**: Methods used to lessen tension, reduce anxiety, and manage pain.

Side effects: Problems caused by a medicine or other treatment. Examples are constipation and drowsiness.

Skin patch: A bandage-like patch that releases medicine through the skin and then into the bloodstream. The medicine enters the blood slowly and steadily.

Standard treatment: The treatment that is accepted and most often used.

Stage: The extent of disease. It can also be a phase of a clinical trial.

Steroids: Medicines that reduces swelling and inflammation.

Stool softeners: Medicine that softens the solid waste in your body, making it easier to pass.

Subcutaneous (sub-kyu-TAY-nee-yus) **injection**: A shot under the skin.

Sublingual: Under the tongue.

Supplements: Vitamins, minerals, herbs, and other things you can take besides medicines.

Tolerance: Occurs when the body gets used to a medicine. The result is that the dose no longer works well. Either more medicine is needed to control the pain or different medicine is needed.

Transcutaneous (tranz-kyu-TAY-nee-yus) **Electrical Nerve Stimulation (TENS)**: A method in which mild electric currents are applied to some areas of the skin by a small power pack connected to two electrodes.

Transmucosal (tranz-myu-KO-sol): Absorbed through the lining of the mouth.

Withdrawal: Signs and symptoms that can appear when long-term use of opioids is stopped or suddenly reduced a lot.

Before You Go to the Pharmacy—Know What You're Getting!

Sometimes people get new prescriptions and are confused about how to take them and when. If your doctor prescribes a new medicine, it's important for you to understand what you will be taking. And as mentioned in chapter 5, get to know your pharmacist. He or she can answer many questions for you.

Before you leave your visit, ask your health care team:

- How do you spell the name of the drug?
- What does the medicine look like? If there is a generic version, does it look the same?
- How many pills (or how much liquid) are in *each* dose?
- How many *times a day* do I take the dose?
- Should I take this medicine with food?
- Can I take it with my other medicine or supplements?

Be sure to read the printed information that comes with your medicine. If you have trouble reading it, ask a friend or family member to read it for you.

In: Coping With Cancer
Editor: Edward H. Ginn

ISBN: 978-1-63321-039-4
© 2014 Nova Science Publishers, Inc.

Chapter 2

EATING HINTS: BEFORE, DURING, AND AFTER CANCER TREATMENT[*]

National Cancer Institute

ABOUT THIS CHAPTER

Eating Hints is written for you—someone who is about to get, or is now getting, cancer treatment. Your family, friends, and others close to you may also want to read this chapter.

You can use this chapter before, during, and after cancer treatment. It has hints about common types of eating problems, along with ways to manage them.

This chapter covers:

- What you should know about cancer treatment, eating well, and eating problems
- How feelings can affect appetite
- Hints to manage eating problems
- How to eat well after cancer treatment ends
- Foods and drinks to help with certain eating problems
- Ways to learn more

---

[*] This is an edited, reformatted and augmented version of National Institutes of Health Publication No. 11-2079, dated January 2011.

Talk with your doctor, nurse, or dietitian about any eating problems that might affect you during cancer treatment. He or she may suggest that you read certain sections or follow some of the tips.

WHAT YOU SHOULD KNOW ABOUT CANCER TREATMENT, EATING WELL, AND EATING PROBLEMS

People with Cancer Have Different Diet Needs

People with cancer often need to follow diets that are different from what they think of as healthy. For most people, a healthy diet includes:

- Lots of fruits and vegetables, and whole grain breads and cereals
- Modest amounts of meat and milk products
- Small amounts of fat, sugar, alcohol, and salt

When you have cancer, though, you need to eat to keep up your strength to deal with the side effects of treatment. When you are healthy, eating enough food is often not a problem. But when you are dealing with cancer and treatment, this can be a real challenge.

When you have cancer, you may need extra protein and calories. At times, your diet may need to include extra milk, cheese, and eggs. If you have trouble chewing and swallowing, you may need to add sauces and gravies. Sometimes, you may need to eat low-fiber foods instead of those with high fiber. Your dietitian can help you with any diet changes you may need to make.

Cancer Treatment Can Cause Side Effects That Lead to Eating Problems

Cancer treatments are designed to kill cancer cells. But these treatments can also damage healthy cells. Damage to healthy cells can cause side effects. Some of these side effects can lead to eating problems.

Common eating problems during cancer treatment include:

- Appetite loss
- Changes in sense of taste or smell

- Constipation
- Diarrhea
- Dry mouth
- Lactose intolerance
- Nausea
- Sore mouth
- Sore throat and trouble swallowing
- Vomiting
- Weight gain
- Weight loss

Some people have appetite loss or nausea because they are stressed about cancer and treatment. People who react this way almost always feel better once treatment starts and they know what to expect.

Things to Do and Think About before You Start Cancer Treatment

- Until treatment starts you will not know what, if any, side effects or eating problems you may have. If you do have problems, they may be mild. Many side effects can be controlled. Many problems go away when cancer treatment ends.
- Think of your cancer treatment as a time to get well and focus just on yourself.
- Eat a healthy diet before treatment starts. This helps you stay strong during treatment and lowers your risk of infection.
- Go to the dentist. It is important to have a healthy mouth before you start cancer treatment.
- Ask your doctor, nurse, or dietitian about medicine that can help with eating problems.
- Discuss your fears and worries with your doctor, nurse, or social worker. He or she can discuss ways to manage and cope with these feelings.
- Learn about your cancer and its treatment. Many people feel better when they know what to expect. See the list of helpful resources in "Ways to Learn More" later in this chapter.

Ways You Can Get Ready to Eat Well

- Fill the refrigerator, cupboard, and freezer with healthy foods. Make sure to include items you can eat even when you feel sick.
- Stock up on foods that need little or no cooking, such as frozen dinners and ready-to-eat cooked foods.
- Cook some foods ahead of time and freeze in meal-sized portions.
- Ask friends or family to help you shop and cook during treatment. Maybe a friend can set up a schedule of the tasks that need to be done and the people who will do them.
- Talk with your doctor, nurse, or dietitian about what to expect. You can find lists of foods and drinks to help with many types of eating problems on later in this chapter.

Not Everyone Has Eating Problems during Cancer Treatment

There is no way to know if you will have eating problems and, if so, how bad they will be. You may have just a few problems or none at all. In part, this depends on the type of cancer you have, where it is in your body, what kind of treatment you have, how long treatment lasts, and the doses of treatment you receive.

During treatment, there are many helpful medicines and other ways to manage eating problems. Once treatment ends, many eating problems go away. Your doctor, nurse, or dietitian can tell you more about the types of eating problems you might expect and ways to manage them. If you start to have eating problems, tell your doctor or nurse right away.

If you start to have eating problems, tell your doctor or nurse right away.

Talk with Your Doctor, Nurse, or Dietitian About Foods to Eat

Talk with your doctor or nurse if you are not sure what to eat during cancer treatment. Ask him or her to refer you to a dietitian. A dietitian is the best person to talk with about your diet. He or she can help choose foods and drinks that are best for you during treatment and after.

Make a list of questions for your meeting with the dietitian. Ask about your favorite foods and recipes and if you can eat them during cancer treatment. You might want to find out how other patients manage their eating problems.

If you are already on a special diet for diabetes, kidney or heart disease, or other health problem, it is even more important to speak with a doctor and dietitian. Your doctor and dietitian can advise you about how to follow your special diet while coping with eating problems caused by cancer treatment.

For more information on how to find a dietitian, contact the American Dietetic Association.

Ways to Get the Most from Foods and Drinks

During treatment, you may have good days and bad days when it comes to food. Here are some ways to manage:

- Eat plenty of protein and calories when you can. This helps you keep up your strength and helps rebuild tissues harmed by cancer treatment.
- Eat when you have the biggest appetite. For many people, this is in the morning. You might want to eat a bigger meal early in the day and drink liquid meal replacements later on.
- Eat those foods that you can, even if it is only one or two items. Stick with these foods until you are able to eat more. You might also drink liquid meal replacements for extra calories and protein.
- Do not worry if you cannot eat at all some days. Spend this time finding other ways to feel better, and start eating when you can. Tell your doctor if you cannot eat for more than 2 days.
- Drink plenty of liquids. It is even more important to get plenty to drink on days when you cannot eat. Drinking a lot helps your body get the liquid it needs. Most adults should drink 8 to 12 cups of liquid a day. You may find this easier to do if you keep a water bottle nearby.
- If others are making meals for you, be sure to tell them your needs and concerns.

Taking Special Care with Food to Avoid Infections

Some cancer treatments can make you more likely to get infections. When this happens, you need to take special care in the way you handle and prepare food. Here are some ways:

- Keep hot foods hot and cold foods cold. Put leftovers in the refrigerator as soon as you are done eating.
- Scrub all raw fruits and vegetables before you eat them. Do not eat foods (like raspberries) that cannot be washed well. You should scrub fruits and vegetable that have rough surfaces, such as melons, before you cut them.
- Wash your hands, knives, and counter tops before and after you prepare food. This is most important when preparing raw meat, chicken, turkey, and fish.
- Use one cutting board for meat and one for fruits and vegetables.
- Thaw meat, chicken, turkey, and fish in the refrigerator or defrost them in the microwave. Do not leave them sitting out.
- Cook meat, chicken, turkey, and eggs thoroughly. Meats should not have any pink inside. Eggs should be hard, not runny.
- Do not eat raw fish or shellfish, such as sushi and uncooked oysters.
- Make sure that all of your juices, milk products, and honey are pasteurized.
- Do not use foods or drinks that are past their freshness date.
- Do not buy foods from bulk bins.
- Do not eat at buffets, salad bars, or self-service restaurants.
- Do not eat foods that show signs of mold. This includes moldy cheeses such as bleu cheese and Roquefort.

For more information about infection and cancer treatment, see *Chemotherapy and You: Support for People With Cancer*, a book from the National Cancer Institute. You can get it free by calling 1-800-4-CANCER (1-800-422-6237) or online at www.cancer.gov/publications.

Using Food, Vitamins, and Other Supplements to Fight Cancer

Many people want to know how they can help their body fight cancer by eating certain foods or taking vitamins or supplements. But, there are no studies that prove that any special diet, food, vitamin, mineral, dietary supplement, herb, or combination of these can slow cancer, cure it, or keep it from coming back. In fact, some of these products can cause other problems by changing how your cancer treatment works.

Talk with your doctor, nurse, or dietitian before going on a special diet or taking any supplements. To avoid problems, be sure to follow their advice.

For more information about complementary and alternative therapies, see *Thinking About Complementary & Alternative Medicine: A Guide for People With Cancer.* You can get this book free from the National Cancer Institute. Call 1-800-4-CANCER (1-800-422-6237) or order online at www.cancer

Talk with your doctor before going on a special diet or taking any supplements. Some vitamins and supplements can change how your cancer treatment works.

A Special Note for Caregivers

- *Do not be surprised or upset if your loved one's tastes change from day to day.* There may be days when he or she does not want a favorite food or says it tastes bad now.
- *Keep food within easy reach.* This way, your loved one can have a snack when he or she is ready to eat. You might put a snack-pack of applesauce or pudding (along with a spoon) on the bedside table. Or try keeping a bag of cut-up carrots on the refrigerator shelf.
- *Offer gentle support.* This is much more helpful than pushing your loved one to eat. Suggest that he or she drinks plenty of clear and full liquids when he or she has no appetite.
- *Talk with your loved one about ways to manage eating problems.* Doing this together can help you both feel more in control.

For more information about being a caregiver, see W*hen Someone You Love Is Being Treated for Cancer.* You can get this book free from the National Cancer Institute. Call 1-800-4-CANCER (1-800-422-6237) or order online at www.cancer

FEELINGS CAN AFFECT YOUR APPETITE DURING CANCER TREATMENT

During cancer treatment, you may feel:

- Depressed
- Anxious

- Afraid
- Angry
- Helpless
- Alone

It is normal to have these feelings. Although these are not eating problems themselves, strong feelings like these can affect your interest in food, shopping, and cooking. Fatigue can also make it harder to cope.

Coping with Your Feelings during Cancer Treatment

There are many things you can do to cope with your feelings during treatment so they do not ruin your appetite. Here are some ideas that have worked for other people.

- *Eat your favorite foods on days you do not have treatment.* This way, you can enjoy the foods, but they won't remind you of something upsetting.
- *Relax, meditate, or pray.* Activities like these help many people feel calm and less stressed.
- *Talk with someone you trust about your feelings.* You may want to talk with a close friend, family member, religious or spiritual leader, nurse, social worker, counselor, or psychologist. You may also find it helpful to talk with someone who has gone through cancer treatment.
- *Join a cancer support group.* This can be a way to meet others dealing with problems like yours. In support group meetings, you can talk about your feelings and listen to other people talk about theirs. You can also learn how others cope with cancer, treatment side effects, and eating problems. Ask your doctor, nurse, or social worker about support group meetings near you. You may also want to know about support groups that meet over the Internet. These can be very helpful if you cannot travel or there is no group that meets close by.
- *Learn about eating problems and other side effects before treatment starts.* Many people feel more in control when they know what to expect and how to manage problems that may occur.
- *Get enough rest.* Make sure you get at least 7 to 8 hours of sleep each night. During the day, spend time doing quiet activities such as reading or watching a movie.

- *Do not push yourself to do too much or more than you can manage.* Look for easier ways to do your daily tasks. Many people feel better when they ask for or accept help from others.
- *Be active each day.* Studies show that many people feel better when they take short walks or do light exercise each day. Being active like this can also help improve your appetite.
- *Talk with your doctor or nurse about medicine if you find it very hard to cope with your feelings.*

Ways to Learn More

The following groups provide support for people with cancer and their families and friends.

The Cancer Support Community

Dedicated to providing support, education, and hope to people affected by cancer.

Call: 1-888-793-9355 or 202-659-9709
Visit: www.cancersupportcommunity.org
E-mail: help@cancersupportcommunity.org

CancerCare, Inc.

Offers free support, information, financial assistance, and practical help to people with cancer and their loved ones.

Call: 1-800-813-HOPE (1-800-813-4673)
Visit: www.cancercare.org
E-mail: info@cancercare.org

To read more about ways to cope with your feelings, see *Taking Time: Support for People With Cancer*. To learn more about coping with fatigue caused by cancer treatment, see *Chemotherapy and You* and *Radiation Therapy and You*. These books are from the National Cancer Institute. You can get free copies at www.cancer.gov/publications or 1-800-4-CANCER (1-800-422-6237).

Eating Problems At-a-Glance

Below is a list of eating problems that cancer treatment may cause. Not everyone gets every eating problem. Some people don't have any problems. Which ones you might have will depend on the type and doses of treatment you receive and whether you have other health problems, such as diabetes or kidney or heart disease.

Talk with your doctor, nurse or dietitian about the eating problems on this list. Ask which ones might affect you.

Eating Problems
Appetite Loss
Changes in Sense of Taste or Smell
Constipation
Diarrhea
Dry Mouth
Lactose Intolerance
Nausea
Sore Mouth
Sore Throat and Trouble Swallowing
Vomiting
Weight Gain
Weight Loss

Appetite Loss

What It Is

Appetite loss is when you do not want to eat or do not feel like eating very much. It is a common problem that occurs with cancer and its treatment. You may have appetite loss for just 1 or 2 days, or throughout your course of treatment.

Why It Happens

No one knows just what causes appetite loss. Reasons may include:

- The cancer itself
- Fatigue
- Pain
- Feelings such as stress, fear, depression, and anxiety
- Cancer treatment side effects such as nausea, vomiting, or changes in how foods taste or smell

Ways to Manage with Food

- *When it is hard to eat, drink a liquid or powdered meal replacement (such as "instant breakfast").*
- *Eat 5 or 6 small meals each day instead of 3 large meals.* You may find it helps to eat smaller amounts at one time. This can also keep you from feeling too full.
- *Keep snacks nearby for when you feel like eating.* Take easy-to-carry snacks such as peanut butter crackers, nuts, granola bars, or dried fruit when you go out.
- *Add extra protein and calories to your diet.*
- *Drink liquids throughout the day*—even when you do not want to eat. Choose liquids that add calories and other nutrients. These include juice, soup, and milk and soy-based drinks with protein.
- *Eat a bedtime snack.* This will give extra calories but won't affect your appetite for the next meal.
- *Change the form of a food.* For instance, you might make a fruit milkshake instead of eating a piece of fruit.
- *Eat soft, cool, or frozen foods.* These include yogurt, milkshakes, and popsicles.
- *Eat larger meals when you feel well and are rested.* For many people, this is in the morning after a good night's sleep.
- *Sip only small amounts of liquids during meals.* Many people feel too full if they eat and drink at the same time. If you want more than just small sips, have a larger drink at least 30 minutes before or after meals.

RECIPE

To help with appetite loss

Banana Milkshake

1 whole ripe banana, sliced
Vanilla extract (a few drops)
1 cup milk

Put all ingredients into a blender.

Blend at high speed until smooth.

Yield: 1 serving
Serving size:
Approximately 2 cups

If made with whole milk:
Calories per serving:
255 calories
Protein per serving: 9 grams

If made with 2% milk:
Calories per serving:
226 calories
Protein per serving: 9 grams

If made with skim milk:
Calories per serving:
190 calories
Protein per serving: 9 grams

Other Ways to Manage

- *Talk with a dietitian.* He or she can discuss ways to get enough calories and protein even when you do not feel like eating.
- *Try to have relaxed and pleasant meals.* This includes being with people you enjoy as well as having foods that look good to eat.
- *Exercise.* Being active can help improve your appetite. Studies show that many people with cancer feel better when they get some exercise each day.

- *Talk with your nurse or social worker if fear, depression, or other feelings affect your appetite or interest in food.* He or she can suggest ways to help.
- *Tell your doctor if you are having nausea, vomiting, or changes in how foods taste or smell.* Your doctor can help control these problems so that you feel more like eating.

CHANGES IN SENSE OF TASTE OR SMELL

What It Is

Food may have less taste or certain foods (like meat) may be bitter or taste like metal. Your sense of smell may also change. Sometimes, foods that used to smell good to you no longer do.

Why It Happens

Cancer treatment, dental problems, or the cancer itself can cause changes in your sense of taste or smell. Although there is no way to prevent these problems, they often get much better after treatment ends.

Ways to Manage with Food

- *Choose foods that look and smell good.* Avoid foods that do not appeal to you. For instance, if red meat (such as beef) tastes or smells strange, then try chicken or turkey.
- *Marinate foods.* You can improve the flavor of meat, chicken, or fish by soaking it in a marinade. You can buy marinades in the grocery store or try fruit juices, wine, or salad dressing. While soaking food in a marinade, keep it in the refrigerator until you are ready to cook it.
- *Try tart foods and drinks.* These include oranges and lemonade. Tart lemon custard might taste good and add extra protein and calories. But do not eat tart foods if you have a sore mouth or sore throat.
- *Make foods sweeter.* If foods have a salty, bitter, or acid taste, adding sugar or sweetener to make them sweeter might help.

- *Add extra flavor to your foods.* For instance, you might add bacon bits or onion to vegetables or use herbs like basil, oregano, and rosemary. Use barbecue sauce on meat and chicken.
- *Avoid foods and drinks with smells that bother you.* Here are some ways to help reduce food smells:
  - Serve foods at room temperature
  - Keep foods covered
  - Use cups with lids (such as travel mugs)
  - Drink through a straw
  - Use a kitchen fan when cooking
  - Cook outdoors
  - When cooking, lift lids away from you

Eat with plastic forks and spoons if you have a metal taste in your mouth.

Other Ways to Manage

- *Talk with a dietitian.* He or she can give you other ideas about how to manage changes in taste and smell.
- *Eat with plastic forks and spoons.* If you have a metal taste in your mouth, eating with plastic forks and spoons can help. If you enjoy eating with chopsticks, those might help, too. Also, try cooking foods in glass pots and pans instead of metal ones.
- *Keep your mouth clean.* Keeping your mouth clean by brushing and flossing can help food taste better.
- *Use special mouthwashes.* Ask your dentist or doctor about mouthwashes that might help, as well as other ways to care for your mouth.
- *Go to the dentist.* He or she can make sure that your changed sense of taste or smell is not from dental problems.
- *Talk with your doctor or nurse.* Tell them about any changes in taste or smell and how these changes keep you from eating.

Constipation

What It Is

Constipation occurs when bowel movements become less frequent and stools become hard, dry, and difficult to pass. You may have painful bowel movements, feel bloated, or have nausea. You may belch, pass a lot of gas, and have stomach cramps or pressure in the rectum.

Why It Happens

Chemotherapy, the location of the cancer, pain medication, and other medicines can cause constipation. It can also happen when you do not drink enough liquids or do not eat enough fiber. Some people get constipation when they are not active.

Ways to Manage with Food

- *Drink plenty of liquids.* Drink at least 8 cups of liquids each day. One cup is equal to 8 ounces.
- *Drink hot liquids.* Many people find that drinking warm or hot liquids (such as coffee, tea, and soup) can help relieve constipation. You might also try drinking hot liquids right after meals.
- *Eat high-fiber foods.* These include whole grain breads and cereals, dried fruits, and cooked dried beans or peas. People with certain types of cancer should not eat a lot of fiber, so check with your doctor before adding fiber to your diet.

Talk with your doctor before taking laxatives, stool softeners, or any medicine to relieve constipation.

RECIPE

To help relieve constipation

Apple/Prune Sauce

1/3 cup unprocessed bran
1/3 cup applesauce
1/3 cup mashed stewed prunes

Blend all ingredients and store in a refrigerator.

Take 1-2 tablespoons of this mixture
before bedtime, then drink 8 ounces of water.

Note: Make sure
you drink the water,
or else this recipe
will not work
to relieve constipation.

Yield:
16 servings

Serving size:
1 tablespoon

Calories per serving:
10 calories

Other Ways to Manage

- *Talk with a dietitian.* He or she can suggest foods to help relieve constipation.
- *Keep a record of your bowel movements.* Show this to your doctor or nurse and talk about what is normal for you. This record can be used to figure out whether you have constipation.
- *Be active each day.* Being active can help prevent and relieve constipation. Talk with your doctor about how active you should be and what kind of exercise to do.
- *Let your doctor or nurse know if you have not had a bowel movement in 2 days.* Your doctor may suggest a fiber supplement, laxative, stool softener, or enema. Do not use any of these without first asking your doctor or nurse.

DIARRHEA

What It Is

Diarrhea occurs when you have frequent bowel movements that may be soft, loose, or watery. Foods and liquids pass through the bowel so quickly that your body cannot absorb enough nutrition, vitamins, minerals, and water from them. This can cause dehydration (which occurs when your body has too little water). Diarrhea can be mild or severe and last a short or long time.

Why it happens

Diarrhea can be caused by cancer treatments such as radiation therapy to the abdomen or pelvis, chemotherapy, or biological therapy. These treatments cause diarrhea because they can harm healthy cells in the lining of your large and small bowel. Diarrhea can also be caused by infections, medicine used to treat constipation, or antibiotics.

Ways to Manage with Food

- *Drink plenty of fluids to replace those you lose from diarrhea.* These include water, ginger ale, and sports drinks such as Gatorade® and Propel®.
- *Let carbonated drinks lose their fizz before you drink them.* Add extra water if drinks make you thirsty or they cause nausea.
- *Eat 5 or 6 small meals each day instead of 3 large meals.*
- *Eat foods and liquids that are high in sodium and potassium.* When you have diarrhea, your body loses these substances, and it is important to replace them. Liquids with sodium include bouillon or fat-free broth. Foods high in potassium include bananas, canned apricots, and baked, boiled, or mashed potatoes.
- *Eat low-fiber foods.* Foods high in fiber can make diarrhea worse. Low-fiber foods include plain or vanilla yogurt, white toast, and white rice. You can find a list of more low-fiber foods later in this chapter.
- *Have foods and drinks at room temperature, neither too hot nor too cold.*
- *Avoid foods or drinks that can make diarrhea worse.* These include:
    - Foods high in fiber, such as whole wheat breads and pasta
    - Drinks that have a lot of sugar, such as regular soda and fruit punch
    - Very hot or very cold drinks
    - Greasy, fatty, or fried foods, such as French fries and hamburgers
    - Foods and drinks that can cause gas. These include cooked dried beans and raw fruits and vegetables.
    - Milk products, unless they are low-lactose or lactose-free
    - Beer, wine, and other types of alcohol
    - Spicy foods, such as pepper, hot sauce, salsa, and chili
    - Foods or drinks with caffeine. These include regular coffee, tea, some sodas, and chocolate.
    - Sugar-free products that are sweetened with xylitol or sorbitol. These are found mostly in sugar-free gums and candy. Read product labels to find out if they have these sweeteners in them.
    - Apple juice, since it is high in sorbitol
- *Drink only clear liquids for 12 to 14 hours after a sudden attack of diarrhea.* This lets your bowels rest and helps replace lost fluids. Let your doctor know if you have sudden diarrhea.

Ask your doctor or nurse before taking medicine for diarrhea.

Other Ways to Manage

- *Talk with a dietitian.* He or she can help you choose foods to prevent dehydration. The dietitian can also tell you which foods are good to eat and which ones to avoid when you have diarrhea.
- *Be gentle when wiping yourself after a bowel movement.* Instead of toilet paper, clean yourself with wet wipes or squirt water from a spray bottle. Tell your doctor or nurse if your rectal area is sore or bleeds or if you have hemorrhoids.
- *Tell your doctor if you have had diarrhea for more than 24 hours.* He or she also needs to know if you have pain and cramping. Your doctor may prescribe medicine to help control these problems. You may also need IV fluids to replace lost water and nutrients. This means you will receive the fluids through a needle inserted into a vein. Do not take medicine for diarrhea without first asking your doctor or nurse.

DRY MOUTH

What It Is

Dry mouth occurs when you have less saliva than you used to. This can make it harder to talk, chew, and swallow food. Dry mouth can also change the way food tastes.

Why It Happens

Chemotherapy and radiation therapy to the head or neck area can damage the glands that make saliva. Biological therapy and some medicines can also cause dry mouth.

Ways to Manage with Food

- *Sip water throughout the day.* This can help moisten your mouth, which can help you swallow and talk. Many people carry water bottles with them.

- *Have very sweet or tart foods and drinks (such as lemonade).* These help you make more saliva. But do not eat or drink anything sweet or tart if you have a sore mouth or sore throat. It might make these problems worse.
- *Chew gum or suck on hard candy, popsicles, and ice chips.* These help make saliva, which moistens your mouth. Choose sugar-free gum or candy since too much sugar can cause cavities in your teeth. If you also have diarrhea, check with your dietitian before using sugar-free products as some sweeteners can make it worse.
- *Eat foods that are easy to swallow.* Try pureed cooked foods or soups. You can find a list of foods and drinks that are easy to chew and swallow later in this chapter.
- *Moisten food with sauce, gravy, or salad dressing.* This helps make food easy to swallow.
- *Do not drink beer, wine, or any type of alcohol.* These can make your mouth even drier.
- *Avoid foods that can hurt your mouth.* This includes foods that are very spicy, sour, salty, hard, or crunchy.

Other Ways to Manage

- *Talk with a dietitian.* He or she can discuss ways to eat even when a dry mouth makes it hard for you to chew.
- *Keep your lips moist with lip balm.*
- *Rinse your mouth every 1 to 2 hours.* Mix 1/4 teaspoon baking soda and 1/8 teaspoon salt with 1 cup warm water. Rinse with plain water after using this mixture.
- *Do not use mouthwash that has alcohol.* Alcohol makes a dry mouth worse.
- *Do not use tobacco products, and avoid second-hand smoke.* Tobacco products and smoke can hurt your mouth and throat.
- *Talk with your doctor or dentist.* Ask about artificial saliva or other products to coat, protect, and moisten your mouth and throat. These products can help with severe dry mouth.

Ways to Learn More

National Oral Health Information Clearinghouse
A service of the National Institute of Dental and Craniofacial Research that provides oral health information for special care patients. Ask about their booklets, *Chemotherapy and Your Mouth* and *Head and Neck Radiation Treatment and Your Mouth.*

Call: 301-402-7364
Visit: www.nidcr.nih.gov
E-mail: nidcrinfo@mail.nih.gov

LACTOSE INTOLERANCE

What It Is

Lactose intolerance occurs when your body cannot digest or absorb a milk sugar called lactose. Lactose is in milk products such as cheese, ice cream, and pudding. Symptoms of lactose intolerance can be mild or severe and may include gas, cramps, and diarrhea. These symptoms may last for weeks or even months after treatment ends. Sometimes, lactose intolerance is a life-long problem.

Why It Happens

Lactose intolerance can be caused by radiation therapy to the abdomen or pelvis or other treatments that affect the digestive system, such as surgery or antibiotics.

Ways to Manage with Food

- *Prepare your own low-lactose or lactose-free foods.*
- *Choose lactose-free or low-lactose milk products.* Most grocery stores have products (such as milk and ice cream) labeled "lactose-free" or "low-lactose."

- *Try products made with soy or rice (such as soy or rice milk and ice cream).* These products do not have any lactose. People with certain types of cancer may not be able to eat soy products. So, ask your dietitian if soy is safe for you to add to your diet.
- *Choose milk products that are low in lactose.* Hard cheeses (such as cheddar) and yogurt are less likely to cause problems.

RECIPE

To help with lactose intolerance

Lactose-Free Double Chocolate Pudding

2 squares baking chocolate (1 ounce each)
1 cup nondairy creamer, rice, soy, or lactose-free milk
1 tablespoon cornstarch
¼ cup granulated sugar
1 teaspoon vanilla extract

Melt chocolate in a small pan.
Measure cornstarch and sugar into a separate saucepan.
Add part of the liquid and stir until cornstarch dissolves.
Add the rest of the liquid.
Cook over medium heat until warm.
Stir in chocolate until mixture is thick and comes to a boil.
Remove from heat.
Blend in vanilla and cool.

Yield:
2 servings
Serving size:
¾ cup
Calories per serving:
382 calories
Protein per serving:
1 gram

Other Ways to Manage

- Talk with a dietitian. He or she can help you choose foods that are low in lactose.

- Talk with your doctor. He or she may suggest medicine to help with lactose intolerance. These include lactase tablets. Lactase is a substance that breaks down lactose.

NAUSEA

What It Is

Nausea occurs when you feel queasy or sick to your stomach. It may be followed by vomiting (throwing up), but not always. Nausea can keep you from getting the food and nutrients you need. Not everyone gets nausea and those who do may get it right after a treatment or up to 3 days later. Nausea almost always goes away once treatment ends.

Why It Happens

Nausea can be a side effect of surgery, chemotherapy, biological therapy, and radiation therapy to the abdomen, small intestine, colon, or brain. It can also be caused by certain types of cancer or other illnesses.

Ways to Manage with Food

- *Eat foods that are easy on your stomach.* These include white toast, plain or vanilla yogurt, and clear broth. Try lemon, lime, or other tart-flavored foods.
- *Eat 5 or 6 small meals each day instead of 3 large meals.* Many people find it easier to eat smaller amounts, more often.
- *Do not skip meals and snacks.* Even if you do not feel hungry, you should still eat. For many people, having an empty stomach makes nausea worse.
- *Choose foods that appeal to you.* Do not force yourself to eat any food that makes you feel sick. At the same time, do not eat your favorite foods, so you don't link them to feeling sick.
- *Sip only small amounts of liquids during meals.* Many people feel full or bloated if they eat and drink at the same time.

- *Have liquids throughout the day.* Drink slowly. Sip liquids through a straw. Or, drink from a water bottle.
- *Have foods and drinks that are not too hot and not too cold.* Let hot foods and drinks cool down and cold foods and drinks warm up before you eat or drink them. You can cool hot foods and drinks by adding ice or warm up cold foods in a microwave.
- *Eat dry toast or crackers before getting out of bed if you have nausea in the morning.*
- *Plan when it is best for you to eat and drink.* Some people feel better when they eat a light meal or snack before treatment. Others feel better when they have treatment on an empty stomach (nothing to eat or drink for 2 to 3 hours before).

Be sure to tell your doctor or nurse if antinausea medicine does not help.

Other Ways to Manage

- *Talk with your doctor about medicine to prevent nausea* (antiemetics or antinausea medicines). Be sure to tell your doctor or nurse if the medicines are not helping. If one medicine does not work well, your doctor may prescribe another. You may need to take them 1 hour before each treatment and for a few days after. The type of cancer treatment you get and how you react to it affects how long you need to take these medicines.
  Acupuncture may also help. Talk with your doctor or nurse if you want to try it.
- *Talk with a dietitian about ways to get enough to eat even if you have nausea.*
- *Relax before each cancer treatment.* You may feel better if you try deep breathing, meditation, or prayer. Many people relax with quiet activities such as reading or listening to music.
- *Rest after meals.* But do so sitting up, not lying down.
- *Wear clothes that are comfortable and loose.*
- *Keep a record of when you feel nausea and why.* Show this to your nurse, doctor, or dietitian. He or she might suggest ways to change your diet.

- *Avoid strong food and drink smells.* These include foods that are being cooked, coffee, fish, onions, and garlic. Ask a friend or family member to cook for you to help avoid cooking smells.
- *Open a window or turn on a fan if your living area feels stuffy.* Fresh air can help relieve nausea. Be sure not to eat in rooms that are too warm or stuffy.

SORE MOUTH

What It Is

Radiation therapy to the head or neck, chemotherapy, and biological therapy can cause mouth sores (little cuts or ulcers in your mouth) and tender gums. Dental problems or mouth infections, such as thrush, can also make your mouth sore.

Why It Happens

Cancer treatments can harm the fast-growing cells in the lining of your mouth and lips. Your mouth and gums will most likely feel better once cancer treatment ends.

Ways to Manage with Food

- *Choose foods that are easy to chew.* Certain foods can hurt a sore mouth and make it harder to chew and swallow. To help, choose soft foods such as milkshakes, scrambled eggs, and custards.
- *Cook foods until they are soft and tender.*
- *Cut food into small pieces.* You can also puree foods using a blender or food processor.
- *Drink with a straw.* This can help push the drinks beyond the painful parts of your mouth.
- *Use a very small spoon* (such as a baby spoon). This will help you take smaller bites, which may be easier to chew.
- *Eat cold or room-temperature food.* Your mouth may hurt more if food is too hot.

- *Suck on ice chips.* Ice may help numb and soothe your mouth.
- *Avoid certain foods and drinks when your mouth is sore.* These include:
  - Citrus fruits and juices, such as oranges, lemons, and lemonade
  - Spicy foods, such as hot sauces, curry dishes, salsa, and chili peppers
  - Tomatoes and ketchup
  - Salty foods
  - Raw vegetables
  - Sharp, crunchy foods, such as granola, crackers, and potato and tortilla chips
  - Drinks that contain alcohol

If you have a sore mouth, do not use tobacco products or drink alcohol.

Other Ways to Manage

- *Talk with a dietitian.* He or she can help you choose foods that are easy on a sore mouth.
- *Visit a dentist at least 2 weeks before starting biological therapy, chemotherapy, or radiation therapy to the head or neck.* It is important to have a healthy mouth before starting cancer treatment. Try to get all needed dental work done before your treatment starts. If you can't, ask your doctor or nurse when it will be safe to go to the dentist. Tell your dentist that you have cancer and the type of treatment you are getting.
- *Rinse your mouth 3 to 4 times a day.* Mix 1/4 teaspoon baking soda and $1/8$ teaspoon salt with 1 cup warm water. Rinse with plain water after using this mixture.
- *Check each day for any sores, white patches, or puffy and red areas in your mouth.* This way, you can see or feel problems as soon as they start. Tell your doctor if you notice these changes.
- *Do not use items that can hurt or burn your mouth, such as*:
  - Mouthwash with alcohol in it
  - Toothpicks or other sharp objects
  - Cigarettes, cigars, or other tobacco products
  - Beer, wine, liquor, or other type of alcohol

- *Tell your doctor and dentist if your mouth or gums are sore.* They can figure out whether these are from treatment or dental problems. Ask the dentist about special products to clean and soothe sore teeth and gums.
- *Ask your doctor about medicine for pain.* He or she may suggest lozenges or sprays that numb your mouth while eating.

RECIPE

To help with a sore mouth

Fruit and Cream

1 cup whole milk
1 cup vanilla ice cream or frozen yogurt
1 cup canned fruit (peaches, apricots, pears) in heavy syrup with juice
Almond or vanilla extract to taste

Blend ingredients in a blender and chill well before serving.

Yield:
2 servings

Serving size:
1½ cups

If made with ice cream:
Calories per serving:
302 calories
Protein per serving:
7 grams

If made with frozen yogurt:
Calories per serving:
268 calories
Protein per serving:
9 grams

Ways to Learn More

National Oral Health Information Clearinghouse
A service of the National Institute of Dental and Craniofacial Research that provides oral health information for special care patients. Ask about their booklets, *Chemotherapy and Your Mouth* and *Head and Neck Radiation Treatment and Your Mouth*.

Call: 301-402-7364
Visit: www.nidcr.nih.gov
E-mail: nidcrinfo@mail.nih.gov

Smokefree.gov
Provides resources, including information about tobacco quit lines, a step-by-step smoking cessation guide, and publications to help you or someone you care about quit smoking.

Call: 1-877-44U-QUIT (1-877-448-7848)
Visit: www.smokefree.gov

SORE THROAT AND TROUBLE SWALLOWING

What It Is

Chemotherapy and radiation therapy to the head and neck can make the lining of your throat inflamed and sore (esophagitis). It may feel as if you have a lump in your throat or that your chest or throat is burning. You may also have trouble swallowing. These problems may make it hard to eat and cause weight loss.

Why It Happens

Some types of chemotherapy and radiation to the head and neck can harm fast-growing cells, such as those in the lining of your throat. Your risk for a sore throat, trouble swallowing, or other throat problems depends on:

- How much radiation you are getting
- If you are getting chemotherapy and radiation therapy at the same time
- Whether you use tobacco or drink alcohol during your course of cancer treatment

Ways to Manage with Food

- *Eat 5 or 6 small meals each day instead of 3 large meals.* You may find it easier to eat a smaller amount of food at one time.
- *Choose foods that are easy to swallow.* Some foods are hard to chew and swallow. To help, choose soft foods such as milkshakes, scrambled eggs, and cooked cereal.
- *Choose foods and drinks that are high in protein and calories.*
- *Cook foods until they are soft and tender.*
- *Cut food into small pieces.* You can also puree foods using a blender or food processor.
- *Moisten and soften foods with gravy, sauces, broth, or yogurt.*
- *Sip drinks through a straw.* This may make them easier to swallow.
- *Do not eat or drink things that can burn or scrape your throat, such as*:
    - Hot foods and drinks
    - Spicy foods
    - Foods and juices that are high in acid, such as tomatoes, oranges, and lemonade
    - Sharp, crunchy foods, such as potato and tortilla chips
    - Drinks that contain alcohol

Tell your doctor or nurse if you:

- Have trouble swallowing
- Feel as if you are choking
- Cough while eating or drinking

Other Ways to Manage

- *Talk with a dietitian.* He or she can help you choose foods that are easy to swallow.
- *Sit upright and bend your head slightly forward when eating or drinking.* Stay sitting or standing upright for at least 30 minutes after eating.
- *Do not use tobacco products.* These include cigarettes, pipes, cigars, and chewing tobacco. All of these can make your throat problems worse.
- *Think about tube feedings.* Sometimes, you may not be able to eat enough to stay strong and a feeding tube may be a good option. Your doctor or dietitian will discuss this with you if he or she thinks it will help you.
- *Talk with your doctor or nurse.* Tell your doctor or nurse if you have trouble swallowing, feel as if you are choking, cough while eating or drinking, or notice other throat problems. Also mention if you have pain or are losing weight. Your doctor may prescribe medicines to help relieve these symptoms. They include antacids and medicines to coat your throat and control your pain.

Ways to Learn More

Smokefree.gov
Provides resources, including information about tobacco quit lines, a step-by-step smoking cessation guide, and publications to help you or someone you care about quit smoking.

Call: 1-877-44U-QUIT (1-877-448-7848)
Visit: www.smokefree.gov

VOMITING

What It Is

Vomiting is another way to say "throwing up."

Why It Happens

Vomiting may follow nausea and be caused by cancer treatment, food odors, motion, an upset stomach, or bowel gas. Some people vomit when they are in places (such as hospitals) that remind them of cancer. Vomiting, like nausea, can happen right after treatment or 1 or 2 days later. You may also have dry heaves, which occur when your body tries to vomit even though your stomach is empty.

Biological therapy, some types of chemotherapy, and radiation therapy to the abdomen, small intestine, colon, or brain can cause nausea, vomiting, or both. Often, this happens because these treatments harm healthy cells in your digestive track.

Ways to Manage with Food

- *Do not have anything to eat or drink until your vomiting stops.*
- *Once the vomiting stops, drink small amounts of clear liquids (such as water or bouillon).* Be sure to start slowly and take little sips at a time.
- *Once you can drink clear liquids without vomiting, try full-liquid foods and drinks or those that are easy on your stomach.* You can slowly add back solid foods when you start feeling better.
- *Eat 5 or 6 small meals each day instead of 3 large meals.* Once you start eating, it may be easier to eat smaller amounts at a time. Do not eat your favorite foods at first, so that you do not begin to dislike them.

Be sure to tell your doctor or nurse if your antinausea medicine is not helping.

Other Ways to Manage

- *Talk with a dietitian.* He or she can suggest foods to eat once your vomiting stops.
- *Ask your doctor to prescribe medicine to prevent or control vomiting* (antiemetics or antinausea medicines). Be sure to tell your doctor or nurse if the medicine is not helping. Your doctor may prescribe another. You may need to take these medicines 1 hour before each

treatment and for a few days after. The type of cancer treatment you get and how you react to it affects how long you need to take these medicines. You may also want to talk with your doctor or nurse about acupuncture. It might also help.

- *Prevent nausea.* One way to prevent vomiting is to prevent nausea.
- *Call your doctor if your vomiting is severe or lasts for more than 1 or 2 days.* Vomiting can lead to dehydration (which occurs when your body does not have enough water). Your doctor needs to know if you cannot keep liquids down.

WEIGHT GAIN

What It Is

Weight gain occurs when you have an increase in body weight. Many people with cancer think they will lose weight and are surprised, and sometimes upset, when they gain weight.

Why It Happens

Weight gain can happen for many reasons:

- People with certain types of cancer are more likely to gain weight.
- Hormone therapy, certain types of chemotherapy, and medicines such as steroids can cause weight gain. These treatments can also cause your body to retain water, which makes you feel puffy and gain weight.
- Some treatments can also increase your appetite so you feel hungry and eat more. You gain weight when you eat more calories than your body needs.
- Cancer and its treatments can cause fatigue and changes in your schedule that may lead to a decrease in activity. Being less active can cause weight gain.

Do not go on a diet to lose weight before talking with your doctor about it. He or she will help figure out why you are gaining weight and discuss what you can do about it.

Ways to Manage with Food

- *Eat lots of fruits and vegetables.* These are high in fiber and low in calories. They can help you feel full without adding a lot of calories.
- *Eat foods that are high in fiber, such as whole grain breads, cereals, and pasta.* People with certain types of cancer should not eat a lot of fiber, so check with your doctor before adding fiber to your diet.
- *Choose lean meats, such as lean beef, pork trimmed of fat, or poultry without skin.*
- *Choose low-fat milk products.* These include low-fat or non-fat yogurt and skim or 1% milk.
- *Eat less fat.* Eat only small amounts of butter, mayonnaise, desserts, fried foods, and other high-calorie foods.
- *Cook with low-fat methods, such as broiling, steaming, grilling, or roasting.*
- *Eat small portion sizes.* When you eat out, take half of your meal home to eat later.
- *Eat less salt.* This helps you not retain water if your weight gain is from fluid retention.

Other Ways to Manage

- *Talk with a dietitian.* He or she can discuss ways to limit the amount of salt you eat if your weight gain is from fluid retention. A dietitian can also help you choose healthy foods and make healthy changes to your favorite recipes.
- *Exercise each day.* Not only does exercise help you burn calories, but studies show that it helps people with cancer feel better. Talk with your doctor or nurse about how much exercise to do while having cancer treatment.
- *Talk with your doctor before going on a diet to lose weight.* He or she can help figure out why you are gaining weight and prescribe medicine (called a diuretic) if you have fluid retention.

WEIGHT LOSS

What It Is

Weight loss is when you have a decrease in body weight.

Why It Happens

Weight loss can be caused by cancer itself, or by side effects of cancer treatment, such as nausea and vomiting. Stress and worry can also cause weight loss. Many people with cancer have weight loss during treatment.

Ways to Manage with Food

- *Eat when it is time to eat, rather than waiting until you feel hungry.* You still need to eat even if you do not feel hungry while being treated for cancer.
- *Eat 5 or 6 small meals each day instead of 3 large meals.* You may find it easier to eat smaller amounts at one time.
- *Eat foods that are high in protein and calories.* You can also add protein and calories to other foods.
- *Drink milkshakes, smoothies, juices, or soups if you do not feel like eating solid foods.* These can provide the protein, vitamins, and calories your body needs.
- *Cook with protein-fortified milk.* You can use protein-fortified milk (instead of regular milk) when cooking foods such as macaroni and cheese, pudding, cream sauce, mashed potatoes, cocoa, soups, or pancakes.

Other Ways to Manage

- *Talk with a dietitian.* He or she can give you ideas about how to maintain or regain your weight. This includes choosing foods that are high in protein and calories and adapting your favorite recipes.

- *Be as active as you can.* You might have more appetite if you take a short walk or do other light exercise. Studies show that many people with cancer feel better when they exercise each day.
- *Think about tube feedings.* Sometimes, you may not be able to eat enough to stay strong and a feeding tube may be a good option. Your doctor or dietitian will discuss this with you if he or she thinks it will help you.
- *Tell your doctor if you are having eating problems, such as nausea, vomiting, or changes in how foods taste and smell.* He or she can help control these so you can eat better.

RECIPES

To help with weight loss

Protein-Fortified Milk

1 quart (4 cups) whole milk

1 cup nonfat instant dry milk

Pour liquid milk into a deep bowl.

Add dry milk and beat slowly with a mixer until dry milk is dissolved (usually less than five minutes).

Refrigerate and serve cold.

Note: If it tastes too strong, start with ½ cup of dry milk powder and slowly work up to 1 cup.

Yield: 1 quart

Serving size: 1 cup

Calories per serving: 211 calories

Protein per serving: 14 grams

High-Protein Milkshake

1 cup protein-fortified milk

2 tablespoons butterscotch sauce, chocolate sauce, or your favorite fruit syrup or sauce

½ cup ice cream

½ teaspoon vanilla extract

Put all ingredients in a blender.

Blend at low speed for 10 seconds.

Yield: 1 serving

Serving size: Approximately 1½ cups

Calories per serving: 425 calories

Protein per serving: 17 grams

Peanut Butter Snack Spread

1 tablespoon nonfat instant dry milk

1 tablespoon honey

1 teaspoon water

5 tablespoons smooth peanut butter

1 teaspoon vanilla extract

Combine dry milk, water, and vanilla, and stir to moisten.

Add honey and peanut butter, and stir slowly until blended

Spread on crackers.

Mixture also can be formed into balls, chilled, and eaten as candy.

Keeps well in a refrigerator, but is hard to spread when cold.

Yield: 6 tbsp

Serving size: 3 tbsp

Calories per serving: 279 calories

Protein per serving: 11 grams

AFTER CANCER TREATMENT

Many Eating Problems Go Away When Treatment Ends

Once you finish cancer treatment, many of your eating problems will get better. Some eating problems, such as weight loss and changes in taste or smell, may last longer than your course of treatment. If you had treatment for head and neck cancer or surgery to remove part of your stomach or intestines, then eating problems may always be part of your life.

Return to Healthy Eating

While healthy eating by itself cannot keep cancer from coming back, it can help you regain strength, rebuild tissue, and improve how you feel after treatment ends. Here are some ways to eat well after treatment ends:

- Prepare simple meals that you like and are easy to make.
- Cook 2 or 3 meals at a time. Freeze the extras to eat later on.
- Stock up on frozen dinners.
- Make cooking easy, such as buying cut-up vegetables from a salad bar.
- Eat many different kinds of foods. No single food has all the vitamins and nutrients you need.
- Eat lots of fruits and vegetables. This includes eating raw and cooked vegetables, fruits, and fruit juices. These all have vitamins, minerals, and fiber.
- Eat whole wheat bread, oats, brown rice, or other whole grains and cereals. These have needed complex carbohydrates, vitamins, minerals, and fiber.
- Add beans, peas, and lentils to your diet and eat them often.
- Go easy on fat, salt, sugar, alcohol, and smoked or pickled foods.
- Choose low-fat milk products.
- Eat small portions (about 6 to 7 ounces each day) of lean meat and poultry without skin.
- Use low-fat cooking methods, such as broiling, steaming, grilling, and roasting.

Talk with a Dietitian

You may find it helpful to talk with a dietitian even when you are finished with cancer treatment. A dietitian can help you return to healthy eating or discuss ways to manage any lasting eating problems.

EATING PROBLEMS THAT MAY BE CAUSED BY CERTAIN CANCER TREATMENTS

Cancer Treatment	What Sometimes Happens: Side Effects
Surgery	• Surgery may slow digestion (how the body uses food). It can also affect eating if you have surgery of the mouth, stomach, intestines, or throat. • After surgery, some people have trouble getting back to normal eating. If this happens, you may need to get nutrients through a feeding tube or IV (through a needle directly into a vein). Note: Surgery increases your need for good nutrition. If you are weak or underweight, you may need to eat a high-protein, high-calorie diet before surgery.
Radiation Therapy	Radiation therapy damages healthy cells as well as cancer cells. When you have radiation therapy to the head, neck, chest, or esophagus, you may have eating problems such as: • Changes in your sense of taste • Dry mouth • Sore mouth • Sore throat • Tooth and jaw problems • Trouble swallowing When you have radiation therapy to the abdomen or pelvis, you may have problems with: • Cramps, bloating • Diarrhea • Nausea • Vomiting

Cancer Treatment	What Sometimes Happens: Side Effects
Chemotherapy	Chemotherapy works by stopping or slowing the growth of cancer cells, which grow and divide quickly. But it can also harm healthy cells that grow and divide quickly, such as those in the lining of your mouth and intestines. Damage to healthy cells can lead to side effects. Some of these side effects can lead to eating problems, such as: • Appetite loss • Changes in your sense of taste • Constipation • Diarrhea • Nausea • Sore mouth • Sore throat • Vomiting • Weight gain • Weight loss
Biological Therapy (Immunotherapy)	Biological therapy can affect your interest in food or ability to eat. Problems can include: • Changes in your sense of taste • Diarrhea • Dry mouth • Appetite loss caused by flu-like symptoms, such as muscle aches, fatigue, and fever • Nausea • Sore mouth • Vomiting • Weight loss, severe
Hormone Therapy	Hormone therapy can affect your interest in food or ability to eat. Problems can include: • Changes in your sense of taste • Diarrhea

LISTS OF FOODS AND DRINKS

Clear Liquids

This list may help if you have appetite loss, constipation, diarrhea, or vomiting.

Types	Liquids
Soups	Bouillon Clear broth Consommé
Drinks	Clear fruit juices (such as apple, cranberry, or grape)
	Clear carbonated soda or water
	Flavored water
	Fruit-flavored drinks
	Fruit punch
	Sports drinks
	Water
	Weak tea with no caffeine
Desserts and snacks	Fruit ices made without fruit pieces or milk
	Gelatin
	Hard candy
	Honey
	Jelly
	Popsicles
Meal replacements and supplements	Clear nutrition supplements (such as Resource® Breeze,) Carnation® Instant Breakfast® juice, and Enlive!®)

Full-Liquid Foods

This list may help if you have appetite loss, vomiting, or weight loss.

Types	Foods and Drinks
Cereals	Refined hot cereals (such as Cream of Wheat®, Cream of Rice®, instant oatmeal, and grits)
Soups	Bouillon Broth
	Soup that has been strained or put through a blender

Types	Foods and Drinks
Drinks	Carbonated drinks
	Coffee
	Fruit drinks
	Fruit punch
	Milk
	Milkshakes
	Smoothies
	Sports drinks
	Tea
	Tomato juice
	Vegetable juice
	Water
Desserts and snacks	Custard (soft or baked)
	Frozen yogurt
	Fruit purees that are watered down
	Gelatin
	Honey
	Ice cream with no chunks (such as nuts or cookie pieces)
	Ice milk
	Jelly
	Pudding
	Sherbet
	Sorbet
	Syrup
	Yogurt (plain or vanilla)
Meal replacement and supplements	Instant breakfast drinks (such as Carnation® Instant Breakfast®)
	Liquid meal replacements (such as Ensure® and Boost®)
	Clear nutrition supplements (such as Resource® Breeze, Carnation® Instant Breakfast® juice, and Enlive!®)

Foods and Drinks That Are Easy on the Stomach

This list may help if you have nausea or once your vomiting is under control.

Types	Foods and Drinks
Soups	Clear broth (such as chicken, vegetable, or beef)
	All kinds (strain or puree, if needed), except those made with foods that cause gas, such as dried beans and peas, broccoli, or cabbage
Drinks	Clear carbonated drinks that have lost their fizz
	Cranberry or grape juice
	Fruit-flavored drinks
	Fruit punch
	Milk
	Sports drinks
	Tea
	Vegetable juices
	Water
Main meals and other food	Avocado
	Beef (tender cuts)
	Cheese, hard (mild types, such as American)
	Cheese, soft or semi-soft (such as cottage cheese or cream cheese)
	Chicken or turkey (broiled or baked without skin)
	Eggs
	Fish (poached or broiled)
	Noodles
	Pasta (plain)
	Peanut butter, creamy (and other nut butters)
	Potatoes, without skins (boiled or baked)
	Pretzels
	Refined cold cereals (such as corn flakes, Rice Krispies®, Rice Chex®, and Corn Chex®)
	Refined hot cereals (such as Cream of Wheat®)
	Saltine crackers
	Tortillas (white flour)
	Vegetables (tender, well-cooked)
	White bread
	White rice
	White toast

Types	Foods and Drinks
Desserts and snacks	Angel food cake Bananas Canned fruit, such as applesauce, peaches, and pears Custard Frozen yogurt Gelatin Ice cream Ice milk Lemon drop candy Popsicles Pudding Sherbet Sorbet Yogurt (plain or vanilla)
Meal replacements and supplements	Instant breakfast drinks (such as Carnation® Instant Breakfast®) Liquid meal replacements (such as Ensure®) Clear nutrition supplements (such as Resource® Breeze, Carnation® Instant Breakfast® juice, and Enlive!®)

Low-Fiber Foods

This list may help if you have diarrhea.

Types	Foods and Drinks
Main meals and other foods	Chicken or turkey (skinless and baked, broiled, or grilled) Cooked refined cereals (such as Cream of Rice®, instant oatmeal, and grits) Eggs Fish Noodles Potatoes, without skins (boiled or baked) White bread White rice
Fruits and vegetables	Carrots (cooked) Canned fruit (such as peaches, pears, and applesauce) Fruit juice Mushrooms String beans (cooked) Vegetable juice

(Continued)

Types	Foods and Drinks
Snacks	Angel food cake
	Animal crackers
	Custard
	Gelatin
	Ginger snaps
	Graham crackers
	Saltine crackers
	Sherbet
	Sorbet
	Vanilla wafers
	Yogurt (plain or vanilla)

High-Fiber Foods

This list may help if you have constipation or weight gain.

Type	Foods and Drinks
Main meals and other foods	Bran muffins
	Bran or whole-grain cereals
	Cooked dried or canned peas and beans (such as lentils or pinto, black, red, or kidney beans)
	Peanut butter (and other nut butters)
	Soups with vegetables and beans (such as lentil and split pea)
	Whole-grain cereals (such as oatmeal and shredded wheat)
	Whole-wheat bread
	Whole-wheat pasta
Fruits and vegetables	Apples
	Berries (such as blueberries, blackberries, and strawberries)
	Broccoli
	Brussel sprouts
	Cabbage
	Corn
	Dried fruit (such as apricots, dates, prunes, and raisins)
	Green leafy vegetables (such as spinach, lettuce, kale, and collard greens)

Type	Foods and Drinks
	Peas
Potatoes with skins
Spinach
Sweet potatoes
Yams
Snacks	Bran snack bars
Granola
Nuts
Popcorn
Seeds (such as pumpkin or sunflower)
Trail mix

Foods and Drinks That Are Easy To Chew and Swallow

This list may help if you have dry mouth, sore mouth, sore throat, or trouble swallowing.

Types	Foods and Drinks
Main meals and other foods	Baby food
Casseroles
Chicken salad
Cooked refined cereals (such as Cream of Wheat®, Cream of Rice®, instant oatmeal, and grits)
Cottage cheese
Eggs (soft boiled or scrambled)
Egg salad
Macaroni and cheese
Mashed potatoes
Peanut butter, creamy
Pureed cooked foods
Soups
Stews
Tuna salad
Custard

(Continued)

Types	Foods and Drinks
Desserts and Snacks	Flan Fruit (pureed or baby food) Gelatin Ice cream Milkshakes Puddings Sherbet Smoothies Soft fruits (such as bananas or applesauce) Sorbet Yogurt (plain or vanilla)
Meal replacements and supplements	Instant breakfast drinks (such as Carnation® Instant Breakfast®) Liquid meal replacements (such as Ensure®) Clear nutrition supplements (such as Resource® Breeze, Carnation® Instant Breakfast® juice, and Enlive!®)

Quick and Easy Snacks

This list may help if you have appetite loss.

Types of Foods and Drinks	Examples
Drinks	Chocolate milk Instant breakfast drinks Juices Milk Milkshakes
Main meals and other foods	Bread Cereal Cheese, hard or semisoft Crackers Cream soups Hard-boiled and deviled eggs Muffins Nuts

Types of Foods and Drinks	Examples
	Peanut butter (and other nut butters)
	Pita bread and hummus
	Pizza
	Sandwiches
Fruits and vegetables	Applesauce
	Fresh or canned fruit
	Vegetables (raw or cooked)
Desserts and snacks	Cakes and cookies made with whole grains, fruits, nuts, wheat germ, or granola
	Custard
	Dips made with cheese, beans, or sour cream
	Frozen yogurt
	Gelatin
	Granola
	Granola bars
	Ice cream
	Nuts
	Popcorn
	Popsicles
	Puddings
	Sherbet
	Sorbet
	Trail mix
	Yogurt

Ways to Add Protein

This list may help if you have appetite loss, sore throat, trouble swallowing, or weight loss.

Types	How To Use
Hard or semisoft cheese	● Melt on:
	- Sandwiches
	- Bread
	- Muffins
	- Tortillas
	- Hamburgers
	- Hot dogs

(Continued)

Types	How To Use
	- Meats and fish
	- Vegetables
	- Eggs
	- Desserts
	- Stewed fruit
	- Pies
	• Grate and add to:
	- Soups
	- Sauces
	- Casseroles
	- Vegetable dishes
	- Mashed potatoes
	- Rice
	- Noodles
	- Meatloaf
Cottage cheese/ricotta cheese	• Mix with or use to stuff fruits and vegetables
	• Add to:
	- Casseroles
	- Spaghetti
	- Noodles
	- Egg dishes (such as omelets, scrambled eggs, and soufflés)
Milk	• Use milk instead of water in drinks and in cooking
	• Use in hot cereal, soups, cocoa, and pudding
Nonfat instant dry milk	• Add to milk and milk drinks (such as pasteurized eggnog and milkshakes)
	• Use in:
	- Casseroles
	- Meatloaf
	- Breads
	- Muffins
	- Sauces
	- Cream soups
	- Mashed potatoes
	- Macaroni and cheese
	- Pudding

Types	How To Use
	- Custard
	- Other milk-based desserts
Meal replacements, supplements, and protein powder	• Use "instant breakfast powder" in milk drinks and desserts • Mix with ice cream, milk, and fruit flavoring for a high-protein milkshake
Ice cream, yogurt, and frozen yogurt	• Add to: - Carbonated drinks - Milk drinks (such as milkshakes) - Cereal - Fruit - Gelatin - Pies • Mix with soft or cooked fruits • Make a sandwich of ice cream or frozen yogurt between cake slices, cookies, or graham crackers • Mix with breakfast drinks and fruit, such as bananas
Eggs	• Add chopped hard-boiled eggs to salads, salad dressings, vegetables, casseroles, and creamed meats • Make a rich custard with eggs, milk, and sugar • Add extra hard-boiled yolks to deviled egg filling and sandwich spread • Beat eggs into mashed potatoes, pureed vegetables, and sauces. (Make sure to keep cooking these dishes after adding the eggs because raw eggs may contain harmful bacteria.) • Add extra eggs or egg whites to: - Custard - Puddings - Quiches - Scrambled eggs - Omelets - Pancake or French toast batter
Nuts, seeds, and wheat germ	• Add to: - Casseroles - Breads - Muffins - Pancakes

(Continued)

Types	How To Use
	- Cookies
	- Waffles
	• Sprinkle on:
	- Fruit
	- Cereal
	- Ice cream
	- Yogurt
	- Vegetables
	- Salads
	- Toast
	• Use in place of breadcrumbs in recipes
	• Blend with parsley, spinach, or herbs and cream to make a sauce for noodle, pasta, or vegetable dishes
Peanut butter and other nut butters	• Roll bananas in chopped nuts
	• Spread on:
	- Sandwiches
	- Toast
	- Muffins
	- Crackers
	- Waffles
	- Pancakes
	- Fruit slices
	• Use as a dip for raw vegetables
	• Blend with milk and other drinks
	• Swirl through soft ice cream and yogurt
Meat, poultry, and fish	• Add chopped, cooked meat or fish to:
	- Vegetables
	- Salads
	- Casseroles
	- Soups
	- Sauces
	- Biscuit dough
	- Omelets
	- Soufflés
	- Quiches
	- Sandwich fillings
	- Chicken and turkey stuffings

Types	How To Use
Beans, legumes, and tofu	• Wrap in pie crust or biscuit dough as turnovers • Add to stuffed baked potatoes • Add to casseroles, pasta, soup, salad, and grain dishes • Mash cooked beans with cheese and milk

Ways to Add Calories

This list may help if you have appetite loss, sore throat, trouble swallowing, or weight loss.

Types	How To Use
Milk	• Use whole milk instead of low-fat • Put on hot or cold cereal • Pour on chicken and fish while baking • Mix in hamburgers, meatloaf, and croquettes • Make hot chocolate with milk
Cheese	• Melt on top of casseroles, potatoes, and vegetables • Add to omelets • Add to sandwiches
Granola	• Use in cookie, muffin, and bread batters • Sprinkle on: - Vegetables - Yogurt - Ice cream - Pudding - Custard - Fruit • Layer with fruits and bake • Mix with dried fruits and nuts for a snack • Use in pudding recipes instead of bread or rice
Dried fruits (raisins, prunes, apricots, dates, figs)	• Plump them in warm water, and eat for breakfast, dessert, or snack • Add to: - Muffins - Cookies - Breads - Cakes

(Continued)

Types	How To Use
	- Rice and grain dishes - Cereals - Puddings - Stuffings - Cooked vegetables (such as carrots, sweet potatoes, yams, and acorn or butternut squash) • Bake in pies and turnovers • Combine with nuts or granola for snacks
Eggs	• Add chopped hard-boiled eggs to salads, salad dressings, vegetables, casseroles, and creamed meats • Make a rich custard with eggs, milk, and sugar • Add extra hard-boiled yolks to deviled egg filling and sandwich spread • Beat eggs into mashed potatoes, pureed vegetables, and sauces. (Make sure to keep cooking these dishes after adding the eggs because raw eggs may contain harmful bacteria.) • Add extra eggs or egg whites to: - Custards - Puddings - Quiches - Scrambled eggs - Omelets - Pancake or French toast batter

Ways to Learn More

For more resources, see *National Organizations That Offer Cancer-Related Services* at www.cancer. In the search box, type in the words "national organizations." Or call 1-800-4-CANCER (1-800-422-6237) for more help.

National Cancer Institute (NCI)
Find out more from these free NCI services.
Call: 1-800-4-CANCER (1-800- 422-6237)
Visit: www.cancer

Chat: www.cancer
E-mail: cancergovstaff@mail.nih.gov

American Dietetic Association
The nation's largest organization of food and nutrition professionals. They can help you find a dietitian in your area.
Visit: www.eatright.org

American Institute for Cancer Research
Answers questions about diet, nutrition, and cancer through its "Nutrition Hotline" phone and e-mail service. Has many consumer and health professional brochures, plus health aids about diet and nutrition, and their link to cancer and cancer prevention.
Call: 1-800-843-8114
Visit: www.aicr.org
E-mail: aicrweb@aicr.org

The Cancer Support Community
Dedicated to providing support, education, and hope to people affected by cancer.
Call: 1-888-793-9355 or 202-659-9709
Visit: www.cancersupportcommunity.org
E-mail: help@cancersupportcommunity.org

CancerCare, Inc.
Offers free support, information, financial assistance, and practical help to people with cancer and their loved ones.
Call: 1-800-813-HOPE (1-800-813-4673)
Visit: www.cancercare.org
E-mail: info@cancercare.org

National Oral Health Information Clearinghouse
A service of the National Institute of Dental and Craniofacial Research that provides oral health information for special care patients.
Call: 301-402-7364
Visit: www.nidcr.nih.gov
E-mail: nidcrinfo@mail.nih.gov

Smokefree.gov

Provides resources, including information about tobacco quit lines, a step-by-step smoking cessation guide, and publications to help you or someone you care about quit smoking.

Call: 1-877-44U-QUIT (1-877-448-7848)

Visit: www.smokefree.gov

INDEX

A

acetaminophen, 12, 14
acid, 58, 73
acupuncture, 22, 26, 76
adults, 49
advocacy, 34, 35
age, 31
agencies, 32
allergic reaction, 11
alternative medicine, 41
antacids, 74
anticancer drug, 13
antidepressants, 17, 18
antiemetics, 68, 75
anti-inflammatory drugs, 12, 41
anxiety, 22, 24, 25, 42, 55
appetite, vii, 3, 45, 47, 49, 51, 52, 53, 55, 57, 76, 79, 84, 90, 91, 95
arthritis, 13
awareness, 24

B

bacteria, 93, 96
bad day, 49
baths, 23
beef, 57, 77, 86
beer, 13, 19, 64
benefits, 28, 31

biofeedback, 22, 23
biopsy, 4
bleeding, 12, 13
blood, 12, 14, 24, 40, 41, 42
blood flow, 24
blood pressure, 40
bloodstream, 42
body weight, 76, 78
bone(s), 4, 5, 42
bone marrow, 4
bone marrow test, 4
bowel, 5, 15, 59, 61, 63, 75
brain, 19, 67, 75
breathing, 11, 16, 17, 23, 25, 26, 39, 68
burn, 70, 73, 77

C

cabbage, 86
caffeine, 62, 84
calorie, 77, 82
cancer cells, 42, 46, 82, 83
cancer pain, vii, 2, 3, 4, 11, 18, 20, 21, 22, 26, 28
cancer treatment, vii, viii, 2, 10, 22, 27, 28, 45, 46, 47, 48, 49, 50, 51, 52, 54, 61, 68, 69, 70, 73, 75, 76, 77, 78, 81, 82
chee, 42
cheese, 46, 50, 65, 78, 86, 89, 91, 92, 95

chemotherapy, 12, 13, 18, 61, 67, 69, 70, 72, 73, 75, 76
chicken, 50, 57, 58, 86, 95
Chinese medicine, 22
circulation, 23, 38
CIS, 32
clinical trials, 33
cocoa, 78, 92
coffee, 59, 62, 69
colon, 67, 75
communication, 6, 29
community, 28, 33
complex carbohydrates, 81
compression, 5
computer, 7
constipation, 15, 42, 59, 60, 61, 84, 88
cooking, 27, 48, 52, 58, 69, 78, 81, 92, 93, 96
cost, 30, 31, 32
cough, 12, 74
coughing, 5
counsel, 28
counseling, 31, 32, 35
covering, 18
craving, 20, 40
crust, 95
cultural beliefs, 8
cure, 41, 51

D

damages, 5, 41, 82
database, 32, 33
dehydration, 61, 63, 76
dentist, 47, 59, 65, 70, 71
Department of Health and Human Services, 8
depression, 3, 18, 25, 40, 55, 57
diabetes, 49, 54
diarrhea, 17, 61, 62, 63, 64, 65, 84, 87
diet, 46, 47, 48, 49, 51, 55, 59, 66, 69, 77, 78, 81, 82, 97
digestion, 82
directives, 35
discomfort, 5, 22, 38

discrimination, 35
diuretic, 78
dizziness, 11
doctors, vii, 1, 2, 3, 5, 6, 7, 18, 19, 30
dogs, 91
dough, 94, 95
dressings, 93, 96
drug addict, 20
drugs, 4, 6, 11, 12, 13, 14, 16, 17, 18, 19, 20, 32, 40, 41

E

eating problems, vii, viii, 45, 46, 47, 48, 49, 51, 52, 53, 54, 79, 81, 82, 83
education, 34, 35, 53, 97
egg, 93, 96
electric current, 20, 42
electrodes, 42
e-mail, 97
emotional effects, vii
emotional problems, 3, 41
employment, 35
energy, 19, 22, 25, 26, 38, 42
equipment, 16
esophagitis, 72
esophagus, 82
everyday life, 27
evidence, 41
exercise, 25, 26, 34, 38, 42, 53, 57, 61, 77, 79

F

families, 31, 33, 35, 53
family members, 29
fat, 46, 62, 77, 81, 95
fear(s), 6, 27, 47, 55, 57
feelings, vii, 24, 27, 28, 29, 42, 45, 47, 52, 53, 54, 57
fever, 11, 12, 13, 41, 83
fiber, 15, 46, 59, 61, 62, 77, 81
financial, 31, 32, 34, 35, 53, 97
financial planning, 31

fish, 50, 58, 69, 92, 94, 95
flavor, 58
flour, 86
fluid, 77, 78
food, 12, 19, 43, 46, 49, 50, 51, 52, 56, 57, 58, 63, 64, 67, 68, 69, 70, 73, 75, 81, 82, 83, 86, 87, 88, 89, 90, 97
force, 26, 42, 68
fruits, 15, 46, 50, 59, 62, 70, 77, 81, 90, 91, 92, 93, 95
funds, 34

G

gel, 23
genetics, 33
ginger, 62
glasses, 15
gout, 13
granola, 55, 70, 91, 96
gravity, 41
growth, 41, 83
guidance, 27, 34
guilty, 29

H

head and neck cancer, 81
healing, 38
health, vii, 1, 2, 4, 5, 6, 8, 9, 10, 11, 15, 17, 18, 20, 22, 28, 30, 31, 32, 33, 34, 35, 40, 43, 49, 54, 97
health care, vii, 1, 2, 5, 6, 8, 9, 10, 11, 15, 17, 18, 20, 22, 28, 31, 32, 35, 40, 43
health care costs, 32
health care professionals, vii, 35
health insurance, 30, 31, 33
health problems, 6, 54
heart disease, 13, 49, 54
heart rate, 23
heartburn, 12
hemorrhoids, 63
history, 13
hospice, 35

hypnosis, 22, 24, 26

I

ibuprofen, 12, 13, 14, 41
image(s), 24, 38, 40
imagery, 22, 24, 25, 38
income, 31
infection, 12, 47, 50
inflammation, 12, 13, 41, 42
injections, 18
injury, 18
intimacy, 3
issues, 4, 29, 33, 35

J

joints, 42

K

kidney, 13, 31, 49, 54, 88
kidney dialysis, 31
kill, 42, 46
knees, 38

L

lactase, 67
lactose, 62, 65, 66, 67
lactose intolerance, 65, 67
laxatives, 15, 41, 60
lead, 6, 21, 46, 76, 83
learning, 23, 40
legal issues, 35
legs, 36, 38, 39
light, 15, 53, 68, 79
liquids, 15, 18, 31, 49, 51, 55, 56, 59, 61, 62, 68, 75, 76
liver, 12, 13
liver damage, 13
lying, 38, 68

Index

M

machinery, 19
materials, 35
matter, 7, 10
meat, 46, 50, 57, 58, 81, 94
Medicaid, 31, 33
medical, 1, 3, 4, 6, 23, 34, 40, 41
medical care, 1, 40, 41
Medicare, 31, 33
medication, 59
medicine, vii, 1, 2, 4, 6, 7, 8, 9, 10, 11, 12, 13, 14, 15, 16, 17, 18, 19, 20, 21, 22, 23, 25, 26, 28, 30, 31, 32, 35, 36, 40, 41, 42, 43, 47, 53, 60, 61, 63, 67, 68, 71, 75, 78
mental health, 28
messages, 2, 19
milk sugar, 65
mind-body, 25, 26
mold, 50
muscle strain, 4
muscles, 23, 25, 26, 39, 42
music, 23, 25, 26, 39, 68

N

narcotics, 14, 41
National Institutes of Health, 1, 34, 45
nausea, 11, 16, 22, 47, 55, 57, 59, 62, 67, 68, 69, 75, 76, 78, 79, 85
nerve, 18, 19, 41
nervous system, 26, 41
NSAIDs, 12, 13, 41
nurses, vii, 1, 3
nutrients, 55, 63, 67, 81, 82
nutrition, vii, 34, 61, 82, 84, 85, 87, 90, 97

O

OH, 41
opioids, 11, 14, 15, 16, 17, 18, 21, 32, 41, 42
oral health, 65, 72, 97
organs, 5
outpatient, 31
OxyContin®, 14
oysters, 50

P

pain, vii, 1, 2, 3, 4, 5, 6, 7, 8, 9, 10, 11, 12, 13, 14, 15, 16, 17, 18, 19, 20, 21, 22, 23, 24, 25, 26, 27, 28, 29, 30, 32, 34, 36, 37, 38, 39, 40, 41, 42, 59, 63, 71, 74
pain control, vii, 2, 3, 6, 7, 8, 9, 15, 17, 21, 30
pain management, 20
palliative, 3, 11, 35
pasta, 62, 77, 88, 94, 95
patient rights, 33
PCA, 18, 41
pelvis, 61, 65, 82
physical therapist, 1
physical therapy, 26
potassium, 62
potato, 70, 73
poultry, 77, 81, 94
prayer, 68
prescription drugs, 10, 33
prevention, 33, 34, 97
professionals, 1, 33, 97
psychiatrist, 24
psychologist, 24, 52
pumps, 18

Q

quality of life, 22, 41

R

radiation, 5, 18, 19, 42, 54, 61, 63, 65, 67, 69, 70, 72, 73, 75, 82
radiation therapy, 5, 61, 63, 65, 67, 70, 72, 73, 75, 82
reactions, 10
reading, 23, 43, 53, 68
rectum, 12, 18, 59

relaxation, 25, 38, 39
relief, 7, 14, 20, 21, 23, 26, 40, 41
religion, 27
resources, vii, 2, 30, 35, 47, 72, 74, 96, 98
restaurants, 50
rhythm, 39
risk, 47, 72
room temperature, 58, 62
routines, 3
rules, 31

S

safety, 4, 41
saliva, 63, 64, 65
saving lives, 34
sensation, 22, 24
senses, 24
services, 35, 96
shape, 38
shellfish, 50
shortness of breath, 26
side effects, 3, 7, 10, 11, 12, 15, 18, 19, 20, 41, 46, 47, 52, 53, 55, 78, 83
signals, 38
signs, 50
skin, 15, 18, 22, 40, 41, 42, 77, 81, 86
sleeping pills, 17
small intestine, 67, 75
smoking, 72, 74, 98
smoking cessation, 72, 74, 98
snaps, 88
social events, 34
social workers, 1, 3, 28
sodium, 62
softener, 61
solid waste, 41, 42
specialists, 3, 30
spinal cord, 5, 18
spinal tap, 4
spine, 5, 19, 41
spirituality, 27
state(s), 3, 24, 29, 31, 35, 40
steroids, 76
stimulation, 42

stomach, 12, 13, 14, 59, 67, 68, 75, 81, 82
stomach ulcer, 13
stress, 22, 24, 25, 31, 34, 55
subcutaneous injection, 18
sweat, 17
sweeteners, 62, 64
swelling, 11, 13, 18, 42
symptoms, 3, 12, 17, 41, 42, 65, 74, 83

T

technician, 23
techniques, 25, 42
teeth, 39, 64, 71
telephone, 34
temperature, 13, 70
tension, 23, 24, 25, 39, 40, 42
therapeutic touch, 22
therapy, 19, 26, 42, 61, 63, 67, 69, 70, 75, 76, 82, 83
thinning, 14
thoughts, 25, 27, 28
thrush, 69
tin, 18, 22, 40
tissue, 81
tobacco, 64, 70, 71, 72, 73, 74, 98
tofu, 95
training, 35
tranquilizers, 17
treatment, vii, viii, 2, 3, 4, 5, 6, 10, 19, 21, 22, 23, 27, 29, 30, 31, 33, 40, 41, 42, 45, 46, 47, 48, 49, 50, 51, 52, 53, 54, 55, 57, 65, 67, 68, 69, 70, 71, 73, 75, 76, 77, 78, 81, 82
trial, 42
tumor, 4, 5, 19

V

vegetables, 15, 46, 50, 58, 62, 70, 77, 81, 87, 88, 91, 92, 93, 94, 95, 96
vein, 18, 31, 41, 42, 63, 82
vitamins, 50, 51, 61, 78, 81

vomiting, 16, 22, 55, 57, 67, 75, 76, 78, 79, 84, 85

W

walking, 5, 15, 16
water, 15, 23, 49, 61, 62, 63, 64, 68, 70, 75, 76, 77, 84, 92, 95
web, 26, 33
weight gain, 76, 77, 88
weight loss, 72, 78, 81, 84, 91, 95
well-being, 28
wheat germ, 91, 93
wires, 38
withdrawal, 17
withdrawal symptoms, 17
worry, 6, 20, 21, 25, 27, 49, 78

X

x-rays, 42